Uterine Fibroids

Uterine fibroids are the commonest benign tumors of the uterus and pelvis, and are the single most common cause of surgery in women apart from childbirth. As such, this pioneering new book, which compares and contrasts conventional surgical treatments with the rapid emergence of uterine artery embolization as an alternative and less invasive procedure, looks set to provide a turning-point for the future treatment of this condition. A host of international experts from gynecology and interventional radiology have contributed chapters, including one by Dr. Jacques Ravina the pioneer of uterine artery embolization. Although the main focus is on embolization, the book also gives a comprehensive account of the epidemiology, pathology, diagnosis, and management of uterine fibroids, and of conventional treatments such as hysterectomy and myomectomy. This all-inclusive approach makes the book suitable for gynecologists, radiologists, and for all trainees and residents looking after patients with uterine fibroids.

Uterine Fibroids

Embolization and other treatments

Edited by

Togas Tulandi MD, FRCSC, FACOG

Professor of Obstetrics and Gynecology, and the Milton
Leong Chair in Reproductive Medicine, McGill University,
Canada

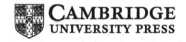

CAMBRIDGE UNIVERSITY PRESS
Cambridge, New York, Melbourne, Madrid, Cape Town, Singapore,
São Paulo, Delhi, Dubai, Tokyo, Mexico City

Cambridge University Press
The Edinburgh Building, Cambridge CB2 8RU, UK

Published in the United States of America by Cambridge University Press, New York

www.cambridge.org
Information on this title: www.cambridge.org/9780521184199

First published 2003
First paperback edition 2010

A catalogue record for this publication is available from the British Library

Library of Congress Cataloguing in Publication data

Uterine fibroids: embolization and other treatments/edited by Togas Tulandi.
      p.   cm.
Includes bibliographical references and index.
ISBN 0-521-81938-5
1. Uterine fibroids–Alternative treatment.   2. Uterine fibroids–Surgery.
3. Women–Diseases–Alternative treatment.   1. Tulandi, T. (Togas)
RC280.U8 U735 2003
616.99′366–dc21   2002034950

ISBN 978-0-521-81938-1 Hardback
ISBN 978-0-521-18419-9 Paperback

Additional resources for this publication at www.cambridge.org/9780521184199

To my family, colleagues, students, and my patients

Contents

Colour plates between pages 48 and 49
(also available at www.cambridge.org/9780521184199)

Contributors

Dr. Haya Al-Fozan
Department of Obstetrics and Gynecology
McGill University
687 Pine Avenue West
Montreal
Quebec H3A 1A1
Canada

Dr. Giovanni Artho
Department of Medical Imaging
McGill University Health Center
1650 Cedar Avenue
Montreal
Quebec H4G 1A4
Canada

Dr. Charles V. Biscotti
Department of Pathology
Cleveland Clinic Foundation
9500 Euclid Avenue
Cleveland
Ohio 44195
USA

Dr. William Brown III
Department of Obstetrics and Gynecology
Mail Code 0660
777 Bannock Street
Denver
Colorado 80204
USA

Dr. L. April Cago
Department of Obstetrics and Gynecology
Wayne State University School of Medicine
Detroit
Michigan 48201
USA

Dr. Charles Coddington III
Department of Obstetrics and Gynecology
Mail Code 0660
777 Bannock Street
Denver
Colorado 80204
USA

Professor Michael Diamond
Department of Obstetrics and Gynecology
Hutzel Hospital
4704 St. Antoine Boulevard
Detroit
Michigan 48201
USA

Dr. Tommaso Falcone
Department of Obstetrics and Gynecology-A81
Cleveland Clinic Foundation
9500 Euclid Avenue
Cleveland
Ohio 44195
USA

Professor Herve Fernandez
Hopital Antoine Beclere
157 Rue de la Porte de Trivaux
92140 Clamart
France

Dr. Amelie Gervaise
Hopital Antoine Beclere
157 Rue de la Porte de Trivaux
92140 Clamart
France

Dr. Jennifer Goedken
Department of Gynecology and Obstetrics
Emory University School of Medicine
69 Butler St SE
Atlanta
Georgia 30303
USA

Dr. Scott Goodwin
Veteran Administration
UCLA Medical Center
Los Angeles
California
USA

Dr. Michael Haggerty
School of Medicine
The University of Pittsburgh
Magee-Womens Hospital
300 Halket Street
Pittsburgh
Pennsylvania 15213
USA

Linda A. Hughes
Holy Cross Hospital
Fort Lauderdale
Florida
USA

Dr. Francis Hutchins Jr.
2170 Chesapeake Harbour
Drive East
Annapolis
Maryland 21403
USA

Dr. Ida Khalili
Department of Medical Imaging
McGill University Health Center
1650 Cedar Avenue
Montreal
Quebec H4G 1A4
Canada

Dr. Wendy J. Landow
Society of Interventional Radiology
Cardiovascular and Interventional Research and Education
Foundation
10201 Lee Highway, Suite 500
Fairfax
Virginia 22030
USA

Dr. Bruce McLucas
UCLA Medical Center
Los Angeles
California 90024
USA

Dr. Camran Nezhat
Department of Gynecology and Obstetrics
Stanford University School of Medicine
Stanford
California
USA

Dr. Caena H. Nezhat
Department of Gynecology and Obstetrics
Stanford University School of Medicine
Stanford
California
USA

Dr. Farr Nezhat
Department of Gynecology and Obstetrics
Stanford University School of Medicine
Stanford
California
USA

Professor Jacques H. Ravina
Service de Gynecologie et Obstetrique
Hopital Lariboisiere
2 Rue Ambroise Pere
75475 Paris Cedex
France

Dr. Caroline Reinhold
Department of Radiology
Montreal General Hospital
1650 Cedar Avenue
Montreal
Quebec H3G 1A4
Canada

Professor John A. Rock
Department of Gynecology and Obstetrics
Emory University School of Medicine
1639 Pierce Drive
Room 4208-WMB
Atlanta
Georgia 30322
USA

Professor Joseph Sanfilippo
School of Medicine
The University of Pittsburgh
Magee-Womens Hospital
300 Halket Street
Pittsburgh
Pennsylvania 15213
USA

Dr. Daniel S. Seidman
Department of Obstetrics and Gynecology
Chaim Sheba Medical Center
Tel Hashomer
and
Sackler School of Medicine
Tel-Aviv University
Tel-Aviv
Israel

Professor Togas Tulandi
Department of Obstetrics and Gynecology
McGill University
687 Pine Avenue West
Montreal
Quebec H3A 1A1
Canada

Dr. Suresh Vedantham
Mallinckrodt Institute of Radiology
Box 8131
510 S Kings Highway
St. Louis
Missouri 63018
USA

Professor George Vilos
Department of Obstetrics and Gynecology
The University of Western Ontario
and
St. Joseph's Health Care
268 Grosvenor St.
London
Ontario N6A 4V2

Dr. Robert L. Worthington-Kirsch
Philadelphia College of Osteopathic Medicine
and
Image Guided Surgery Associates, PC
5735 Ridge Avenue, Suite 106
Philadelphia
Pennsylvania 19128
USA

Preface

Leiomyoma or fibroid is the most common benign tumor occurring in the uterus and in the female pelvis. Fibroids are the primary indication for hysterectomies and represent over 30% of the total number of hysterectomies. There are other treatments of uterine fibroids including expectant management, medical treatment, conservative surgical treatment, and the novel uterine artery embolization. If hysterectomy is indicated, it can also be done by laparoscopy. The book *Uterine Fibroids: Embolization and Other Treatments* has been written to address all these modalities with a special emphasis on the newest treatment – the uterine artery embolization.

The contributors are gynecologists and interventional radiologists who are pioneers in their field and who have many years of experience in the areas they describe. The first nine chapters of the book focus on the epidemiology, diagnosis, histopathology, and the conventional treatments of uterine fibroids. The remaining 10 chapters are dedicated to uterine artery embolization. This second part starts with a history of embolization of uterine myoma written by its pioneer Dr. Jacques H. Ravina. He stated "A new therapeutic approach was born; we have entered an unknown field and began our work as pioneers." Other contributors are those who have popularized this technique worldwide and they discuss the basic, clinical aspects and limitation of uterine artery embolization.

This is a book for students, residents, fellows, gynecologists and radiologists. Information in this book will be helpful in obtaining an understanding of uterine fibroids, to help in consulting patients, and to adopt the technique in the reader's own institution.

The authors is grateful to the contributors and to the staff of Cambridge University Press for their support for this edition of the book and for their expertise in publishing medical works.

Professor Togas Tulandi MD

Foreword

Uterine fibroids have been a major problem for women throughout the centuries manifesting themselves primarily with bladder, bowel, and pressure symptoms relating to their size; and abnormal uterine bleeding and infertility depending upon their location. They have prompted the use of a number of therapeutic approaches including hysterectomy, hysteroscopic surgery, and various laparoscopic approaches including excision, thermogenic, and cryogenic myolysis. The most recent development in the management of uterine fibroids is the use of arterial embolization.

This publication addresses all of the areas in regards to fibroids in an expansive, thorough, and interesting fashion. Chapters include an overview of the incidences of fibroids, and the changing nature as far as treatment is concerned in regards to an aging population interested in fertility. Histopathology is explored, as well as attention to physiology and unicellular origin of fibroids.

Diagnostic imaging, with the appearance of the CAT scan and MRI, has changed the nature of our understanding of myomas in that now penetration into the cavity and other anatomical distortions can be more precisely delineated prior to definitive surgery and/or treatment. The chapter on laparoscopic management includes discussions of all of those techniques that have required an invasive approach in order to manage the patient with symptomatic myomas.

The pregnant patient with myoma represents a special challenge. These myomas may cause premature labor, and are problematic in cesarean sections.

These topics are covered in an interesting contribution. The major question is, should a patient have a myomectomy prior to conceiving or is it worth the risk of allowing time to pass in order to see what manifestations the patient has on fibroids during her pregnancy with severe pain being rare but most common? Expectant management as well as medical management is also addressed. Certainly a good argument is made for these modes of conservative treatment.

The major portion of this text centers on embolization with a thorough discussion of the vascular anatomy. This is almost a "how to book". Certain complications have been noticed after embolization – pain management being the primary one – in the first 24 hours, and the modalities of treatment and an understanding of the path of pathophysiology behind this phenomenon are discussed.

Results of uterine artery embolization are evaluated. In all, the procedure works well but patient selection, as in everything, is critical. Going forward, the future of embolization as a non-invasive technique in the treatment of myomas is discussed together with a consideration of fertility.

This an excellent book. It covers fibroids in depth and provides new insights into their pathogenesis and treatment by describing not only conventional methods of treatment but also uterine artery embolization which is now an option.

Professor Alan H. DeCherney MD

Uterine fibroids: epidemiology and an overview

Jennifer Goedken and John A. Rock

Emory University School of Medicine, Georgia, USA

Prevalence

Leiomyomata, commonly referred to as fibroids, are the most common tumors of the female genital tract. Their prevalence is impossible to fully assess as many do not come to clinical attention. However, rates are frequently stated to be over 40% in women 40 years or older.[1] With more systematic evaluation, higher rates have been noted. Sixty-nine percent of women who underwent a hysterectomy for noncancerous conditions in Maryland, USA, were found to have fibroids, approximately half of which were not suspected prior to surgery.[2]

With scrupulous histologic examination, fibroids were found by Cramer and Patel in 77 of 100 consecutive hysterectomy specimens.[3] Prevalence reported by histology may reflect only those tumors associated with symptoms rather than a true estimation of their occurrence. In fact, histologically confirmed tumors may only represent 29% of patients for whom sonographic evidence of fibroids exists.[4]

In 1998, a study was undertaken to determine the prevalence of occult fibroids in a random sample of premenopausal women using vaginal ultrasonography. A high percentage (62%) of these women were found to have sonographic evidence of fibroids.[5] However, only 5.4% of 335 Swedish women were found to have fibroids on ultrasonographic examination.[6] Additionally, the occurrence was only 10.1% in 11 258 Japanese women.[7] It is clear that though fibroids are a very common pathology, the exact prevalence rate may be impossible to ascertain

and may have some significant ethnic and/or environmental associations.

Perhaps more important than the prevalence, is the extent of morbidity for which fibroids are associated. Uterine fibroids are known to be a cause of symptoms such as abnormal bleeding, pelvic pain, dyspareunia, constipation and urinary frequency. The average annual rate of hospitalization associated with the diagnosis of fibroids from 1989 to 1990 in the United States was 3.0 per 1000 woman-years. Of these, 98% underwent some type of surgery, 83% of which included a hysterectomy.[8]

A review of both prospective[9] and retrospective data[10,11] from the United States shows that fibroids are the primary indication for hysterectomies. This equates to total annual incidence rates of fibroid-related hysterectomy of 1.9–3.6 per 1000 woman-years. These rates have not changed since 1965[12,13] and represent 30.7–33.5% of the total number of hysterectomies. Similar figures have been found in Canada,[14,15] Finland,[16,17] France,[18] Greece,[19] Denmark,[20] and England and Scotland[21] (Table 1.1). With hysterectomy being the most common non-pregnancy related surgical procedure performed on women, fibroids are the single largest cause for surgery in women. Currently, they account for approximately 200 000 hysterectomies performed each year among premenopausal women in the United States.[10,11]

Presumably, women who undergo a hysterectomy represent those with severe fibroid-related symptoms or those who have failed other means of therapy. An assumption can thus be made that most

Table 1.1. Hysterectomies for fibroids

Study	Percentage of hysterectomies	Prevalence rate (per 1000 woman years)
Canada		
Allard & Rochette (1991)[14]	27.2[a] (1988)	1.8[a]
Hall & Cohen (1994)[15]	19–30	1.2–1.9[a]
Finland		
Luoto et al. (1997)[16]	48	3.0[a]
Vuorma et al. (1998)[17]	45 (1987)–47 (1992)	1.6–1.9[a]
France		
Chapron et al. (1999)[18]	34–58	N/A
Greece		
Chryssikopoulos & Loghis (1986)[19]	54.6	N/A
Denmark		
Gimbel et al. (2001)[20]	35 (1988)–37 (1998)	0.7–0.7[a]
England–Scotland		
Vassey et al. (1992)[21]	38.5	2.7

[a]Results extrapolated by this author from unadjusted data provided in these studies.
N/A: not available.

of these women had multiple office visits and medical treatments prior to their hysterectomy.

Demographics

Diagnosis rates of uterine fibroids increase with age through the reproductive years (Figure 1.1)[4,8,10,22] (Figure 1.2).[2,21,23,24,25,26,27] According to most studies, these rates decrease by 42–90% after menopause.[2,22,26,28,29]

Besides one report,[29] most epidemiologic studies reveal that the prevalence of uterine fibroids is higher in black than in white women (Table 1.2).[2,4,9,10,24,27,30] This difference was reported as early as 1894[31]. Although most existing studies report rates based on histology, the difference was also noted incidentally in women randomly recruited to receive vaginal ultrasounds.[5] After adjusting for potential variables, the ratio between black and white women was 3.3–9.4.[4,24]

Black women are diagnosed to have fibroids at a younger age than white women.[4,32] Also, they

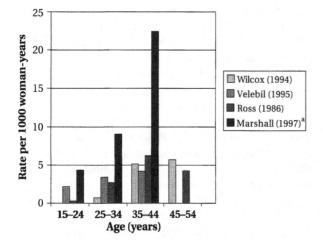

Figure 1.1. Diagnosis rates for fibroids by age (per 1000 woman years).
[a]Diagnosis made by histology, sonography, and physical examination.
In the remaining studies, diagnosis is based on histology only.

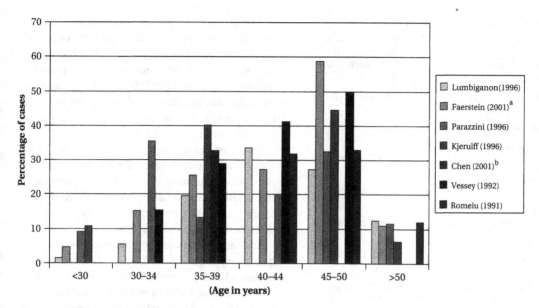

Figure 1.2. Diagnosis rates of fibroids by age (percentage of cases).
[a]Diagnosis made by histology and sonography.
[b]Diagnosis made by visual identification.
In the remaining studies, diagnosis rates were based on histology only.

underwent fibroid-related hysterectomy at an earlier age than white women (41.7 years vs. 44.6 years), their uterine weight was 105.7 g heavier, and the incidence of anemia was higher.[2] Among other ethnic groups, the prevalence of fibroids in Hispanics and Asian women is similar to those of whites.[4] However, as stated previously, studies from both Japan and Sweden, presumably homogenous populations, showed lower rates.[6,7]

Risk factors

Uterine fibroids represent a major public health issue, but there is minimal epidemiological research available on them.[33]

Menstrual history

The growth of fibroids is under the influence of steroid hormones and the rate of diagnosis of fibroid increases during the reproductive years and decreases after menopause. However, a review of consecutive hysterectomy specimens with increased serial sectioning actually revealed the rate of fibroids to be slightly increased in postmenopausal women (84% vs. 74%), but the number and size of the tumors were significantly lower.[3] This represents the limitations of existing studies, that a significant number of asymptomatic fibroids were potentially mislabeled as controls because they do not come to clinical attention.

Some studies have shown that earlier age at menarche increases the risk of fibroids.[23,24,26,29,34,35] This is thought to be secondary to longer exposure to steroid hormones. However, there are no complimentary studies looking at fibroids in relation to age of menopause.

Reproductive history

Parity has been found to be inversely associated with uterine fibroids in most studies,[22,23,25,27,34] but not all.[9,24] The reduction in risk seems to increase with the number of children. The risk of fibroids in women

Table 1.2. Prevalence of fibroids by race

Authors Means of diagnosis	Odds ratio for Black versus White women
Faerstein et al. (2001)[24] Ultrasound/histology	9.4 (CI, 5.7–15.7)
Chen et al. (2001)[27] Visual identification	1.9 (CI, 1.4–2.5)[a]
Kjerulff et al. (1996)[2] Histology	5.6 (CI, 4.0–8.0)[a]
Wilcox et al. (1994)[10] Histology	2.4 (CI, 1.3–4.5)[a]
Marshall et al. (1997)[4] Ultrasound/histology/exam	3.2 (CI, 2.6–4.0)
Brett et al. (1997)[a] Histology	1.9 (CI, 1.3–2.9)
Meilahn et al. (1989)[30] Histology	1.7 (CI, 1.1–2.5)[a]

[a]Odds ratios were calculated by this author using unadjusted data from these studies.
CI: confidence intervals.

with three-term births is reduced by 50–90%.[22,23,24] Of interest, Chen et al. found the same protection that was afforded parous white women was not afforded black women.[27] Some limitations to drawing conclusions from this data include the small number of black women in their study ($n = 70$). Additionally, their definition of parity referred to number of living children and not true parity rates. Finally, their population was women undergoing a tubal ligation. Subsequently, there were a low number of nulliparous women in their study. However, this should actually function to bias the results so that no association is seen. Regardless, their findings bear further investigation because an association between race and parity has not been examined elsewhere.

There has been no association noted with age at first birth and fibroids.[22,23,24,25,26] However, there is conflicting data regarding age at last birth (i.e., time since last birth) as a risk factor. Some studies show no association,[24,25,27,34] while others show a decreased risk with later age at, or less time since, last pregnancy.[22,23] Marshall et al. attempted to address the potential combined effect of both age at first and last delivery on the risk for fibroids. The results from

this large cohort study reveal that earlier age at first birth and increased years since last birth were both risk factors.[4] Another study showed that the protective effect of parity on fibroids was not apparent in women 45 years or older.[25] This may be explained by an underlying increase in risk secondary to longer time since last birth or just longer time of exposure to steroid hormones in general.

Voluntary and spontaneous abortions are not associated with the prevalence of uterine fibroids.[9,23,27] However, in one study there was a 40% decrease in risk of fibroids in women with two or more induced abortions.[25] Again, this finding was only significant in women younger than 45 years of age.

A correlation between infertility and fibroids is frequently reported.[24,25,34] Whether infertility, through decreased parity, is the cause or the result of fibroids is unclear. Also, there is a real potential for selection bias in women with infertility. These women typically undergo more frequent and more extensive pelvic examinations. This may lead to increased incidental detection of fibroids.

There has been a question of whether the association between fibroids and parity can be accounted for by an underlying association with infertility. Marshall et al. evaluated women with a history of infertility and still found that parity was inversely associated with fibroids.[4] It appears that parity provides protection from fibroids. Furthermore, in a recent review of the literature, decreased pregnancy and implantation rates were found in women with submucous fibroids. Excision of fibroids in this location only, improved fertility rates.[24,25]

The specific factors that account for the observed associations between menstrual and reproductive history and fibroids are not certain. Elevated estrogen levels during the reproductive years have been a common hypothesis.[22] Elevated progesterone levels have also been considered.[35] Both hypotheses are supported by the effect seen with gonadotropin-releasing hormone (GnRH) agonists,[36] as well as the antiprogesterone, mifepristone (RU 486),[37] on the growth of fibroids.

Non-hormonal factors may be involved. Increased mitotic activity noted in the myometrium during the luteal phase of the menstrual cycle may be a factor in

Table 1.3. Oral contraceptive use and risk of fibroids

Authors	Risk ratio	Study type Myoma evidence
Royal College of General Practitioners (1974)[41]	0.99 prior use 0.41 ($P < 0.01$) current use	Cohort histology
Ramcharan et al. (1980)[40]	1.5 (CI, 0.9–2.7) ever use	Cohort histology
Ross et al. (1986)[22]	0.64 (CI, 0.48–0.93) within past six months 0.5 ($P = 0.015$, linear trend) 12 years of use	Cohort histology
Parazzini et al. (1992)[28]	1.3 (CI, 0.9–2.0) < three years use 0.8 (CI, 0.5–1.3) ≥ three years use	Case-control histology
Samadi et al. (1996)[29]	1.0 (CI, 0.7–1.6) > three months use	Case-control histology
Parazzini et al. (1996)[25]	1.5 (CI, 1.0–1.9) ever use	Case-control histology
Lumbiganon et al. (1996)[23]	0.76 (CI, 0.66–0.92) ever use	Case-control histology
Marshall et al. (1998)[33a]	1.03 (CI, 0.93–1.15) prior use 0.80 (CI, 0.67–0.94) current use	Cohort histology and sonography
Sato et al. (2000)[34]	1.06 (CI, 0.25–4.17)[a] ever use	Case control histology
Chen et al. (2001)[27]	0.9 (CI, 0.6–1.4) Whites 1.7 (CI, 0.8–3.5) Blacks	Case-control visual identification
Faerstein et al. (2001)[24]	0.7 (CI, 0.5–1.1) prior use 0.2 (CI, 0.1–0.6) current use	Case control history and sonography

[a]Result extrapolated by this author from data provided in this study.
CI: confidence interval.

the induction of fibroids.[33] Indeed, there is more mitotic activity in fibroids of women taking exogenous progestins.[38] Similarly, an increased number of menstrual cycles may lead to an increase in the number of cell divisions that the myometrium undergoes. This could allow for a greater chance of mutation in genes that control myometrial proliferation.[38]

Non-hormonal mechanisms may be involved with the association between parity and fibroids. Myometrial hypertrophy during pregnancy could inhibit the clonal expansion necessary to produce clinically detectable fibroids.[38] Additionally, apoptosis during uterine regression could eliminate or reduce the size of microscopic fibroids.[33] Walker et al. also found a decreased risk of fibroids with parity in an animal model.[39]

Exogenous hormones

Contraceptive

There have been many studies evaluating the relationship between oral contraceptives (OC) and fibroids, but the results have been conflicting. Two studies reveal an increased risk with OC use,[25,40]

three show no association,[27,29,34] and five show a decreased risk[22,23,24,33a,41] (Table 1.3). It appears that the decreased risk is seen only with recent or current use.[22,24,33a,41] One study shows a trend of decreasing risk with increasing duration,[22] while others could not find this association.[28,33a] Overall, this epidemiologic data suggest little to no effect of past OC use, but a potential protective effect of current use.

The primary difficulty with making any inferences from the association of OC use and fibroids is the potential for detection bias. OC use may enhance the diagnosis of fibroids because of more frequent surveillance. A study of the relationship between OC use and fibroids by frequency of Pap (Papanicolaou) smears (i.e. an indicator of medical surveillance) showed increased diagnosis in women using and not using OCs.[29] It has to be noted that current OC use may mask the presence of fibroids by reducing their symptoms.[42] Some clinicians have avoided the use of OC in women with fibroids. This practice may have lead to a decreased association in earlier studies.[43]

Much less is known about other forms of exogenous hormones and their association with fibroids. A study in Thailand showed a significant decrease in the diagnosis of fibroids in women with a history of depot medroxyprogesterone acetate (DMPA) use. This benefit significantly increased with duration of use.[23] However, this finding appears to be in contrast to observations that suggest a stimulatory effect of progestins[35] on fibroids and regression with the antiprogesterone, mifepristone.[37] Explanations may include suppression of the endometrium,[44] a known effect of progestins, or a hypoestrogenic state induced by DMPA use, especially long term.[45]

Hormone replacement

Regression of fibroids is thought to occur after menopause. However, the potential effect of hormone replacement therapy (HRT) on fibroids has not been well studied. Two studies showed increased rates of diagnosis of fibroids and need for treatment in women using HRT.[26,40] However, both of these studies included data from women that may have received HRT in an era when unopposed estrogen was commonly used.

More recently, a study using a depot form of estradiol and prasteronenantate showed a significant increase in the number and size of fibroids with use.[46] Four other studies demonstrated a significant increase in number and/or volume of fibroids in women using percutaneous estrogen formulas, either transdermal estradiol 50 μg/day[47,48,49] or 1 mg estradiol gel.[50] Their regimens included 10 mg of medroxyprogesterone acetate for 12 days a month[47,48,50] or 5 mg continuously.[49] Although these studies showed evidence of fibroid growth, this effect appeared to be self-limited with no further increase noted after 6[48,50] or 12 months.[47]

Another study did not show any increase in fibroid volume with the administration of transdermal estradiol and 5 mg of nomegestrolo acetate daily.[51] The weaknesses of these studies are that none of them had an appropriate control (i.e., placebo) group and they used a high dose of progestin. To address these issues Palomba et al. undertook a prospective study to compare the use of a combination of transdermal estradiol with 2.5 mg medroxyprogesterone acetate daily with placebo. They showed no significant change in the size or number of the fibroids.[52]

There is no evidence of increase in the growth or number of fibroids with oral HRT.[47,49,53] Also, selective estrogen receptor agonists appear to cause a decrease or no change in the size of fibroids.[48,53,54,55] Importantly, even in the studies that showed an increased growth of fibroids with HRT, most women remained asymptomatic.[48,49] On the contrary, there is some data suggesting that submucosal fibroids are associated with abnormal uterine bleeding in women receiving HRT.[56,57]

Finally, there is evidence from two studies that included valid control groups that fibroids did not regress in the placebo group over the one-year course of the studies.[54,55] This brings into question the belief that these tumors regress after menopause. Instead they may not come to clinical attention because they are asymptomatic or were treated premenopausally.

The current data regarding HRT and its potential effect of fibroids is complicated by the various HRT regimens used and frequent lack of controls. More data is needed before any conclusions can be made.

Obesity and smoking

Since experimental data have indicated that the growth of fibroids is dependent on levels of both estrogen and progesterone,[35,58] factors influencing the levels of these hormones might also be important. Obesity, which is known to elevate the level of estrogen through increased peripheral conversion in adipose cells, may be one such factor. Indeed, most studies have shown increased risk of fibroids in the obese (Body Mass Index, BMI > 24).[22,23,24,25,59,60] However, a few have not.[26,27,29] Studies that showed an increase in risk found that effect to be insignificant at the highest levels of BMI.[23,25] One study found that Japanese women with higher body fat despite overall BMI < 24 and those with more upper body fat were at the highest risk.[61] Another study examined the relationship between BMI and uterine weight and found a significant association.

Women who smoke cigarettes behave as though they are relatively estrogen deficient with increased rates of osteoporosis, early menopause and lower rates of endometrial cancer.[62,63] In theory, smoking would lower the risk of fibroids. However, current data are conflicting. Some reported a decrease in risk of 30–50% among smokers[22,23,26,63,64] specifically in current smokers.[63] Others found an increased risk,[27] no effect,[24,59,65] or a protective effect of smoking only in women of low BMI.[29] Perhaps the elevated estrogen production in adipose tissue in obese women outweighs the opposing anti-estrogen effect of smoking. It is also possible that there is a detection bias because these women might seek medical care more often secondary to diseases related to their smoking and obesity.[29]

Miscellaneous

The association between obesity and fibroids raises the question whether other obesity-related factors affect the growth of fibroids. In one study, college athletes and controls were surveyed regarding medical and reproductive history. The self-reported prevalence of fibroids was significantly lower in the athletes compared to their non-athletic counterparts. The authors suggested that this may be due to a decrease in the extraglandular conversion of androgen to estrogen secondary to increased leanness.[65]

Diet is obviously related to obesity. In the only study addressing diet in relation to fibroids, the authors reported a 70% increased risk with frequent consumption of red meat, a 50% reduction with green vegetables, and a 20% reduction with fruit.[64] The associations were significant and independent of other variables. In this study, there was no relationship between BMI and fibroids.[64] Thus the observed dietary associations may reflect nutrients that are etiologically relevant to fibroids. However, it is more likely that they reflect an unmeasured non-dietary lifestyle characteristic.[66]

Uterine irritation has been suggested to play a role in the etiology of fibroids. Potential irritants that have been studied include the use of intrauterine devices (IUD), pelvic inflammatory disease (PID), chlamydial infection and talc use. There appears to be no association between fibroids and the use of IUDs.[22,23,27,34,66a,67] There have only been two studies evaluating the relationship between fibroids and

genital infections. One showed no association.[22] Another study showed an 80% increased risk in women with a self-reported history of PID and a trend toward increasing risk with a number of infections. There was no association between reported chlamydial infection and fibroids.[67] The same study found a fivefold risk of fibroids in women that reported a history of IUD use and a superimposed infection. These findings may be complicated by recall bias because they relied heavily on self-reporting.

The use of perineal talc, a possible irritant, was associated with a 1.7-fold increase in diagnosis rate of fibroids in current users and a 2.1-fold increase in former users. However, this could be secondary to selection bias. Women might use perineal talc due to fibroid-related increased menstrual flow.[67]

The similarities between smooth muscle tumors and atheromatous plaques has lead Faerstein et al. to investigate a possible correlation between atherogenic factors and a risk for fibroids. They found a 2.1-fold increased risk of fibroids in women with hypertension on antihypertensive medication. This association was seen even after adjustment for BMI and race. The risk was strongest in women diagnosed with hypertension prior to 35 years of age, hypertension for at least five years, and on antihypertensive medication for over five years.[67] Similar findings were seen in another study of hysterectomy proven fibroids.[68] However, the retrospective nature of the studies may lead to selection bias because women using more health care services may be more likely to be both diagnosed with hypertension and fibroids. Diabetes, another marker for atherogenesis, has not been shown to be associated with fibroids.[67]

Family history and genetics

Uterine fibroids seem to be more common in women with a positive family history. One study in Thailand found women who reported a family history of fibroids were 3.5 times more likely to have fibroids.[23] A study in Baltimore, USA, revealed a weaker association with a 50% increased risk (Confidence Interval, CI, 0.96–2.41) among women with mothers who had a hysterectomy for fibroids.[24]

Two Russian twin-pair studies alluded to a possible genetic predisposition. Both showed a twofold increase risk of fibroids in women with a sister affected[69] or two first-degree relatives.[70] A Finnish cohort study of twins also found that concordance for being hospitalized for uterine fibroid related morbidity was nearly twice as high in monozygotic than dizygotic twins.[71]

Fifty to sixty percent of uterine fibroids are karyotypically normal. However, aberration involving chromosomes 6,7, 12, and 14 are commonly found.[72] Rearrangements of these chromosomes consistently affect two newly discovered high-mobility group protein genes, HMGIC and HMGIY. They encode proteins that seem to function in architectural transcription and may be involved in the aberrant growth of fibroids.[73] Further discoveries in the area of cytogenetics may provide the explanation for the observed familial tendency of fibroids and the increased prevalence in African-American women.

Future research

Clarifying the etiology, natural history and risk factors associated with fibroids will provide the possibility of preventing and more successfully treating this serious public health problem. Future studies need to take into account the known difficulty with assigning controls in light of the significant amount of subclinical disease. Prospective studies would aid in reducing the amount of selection and recall bias that is inherent in most current studies. Further investigation into hypotheses regarding fibroids and associations with non-hormonal factors such as cellular mitotic activity and apoptosis should be undertaken. Finally, more investigation into the cytogenetic and molecular aspects of fibroids may eventually lead to defining genetic loci that are important in the induction of these tumors.

REFERENCES

1. Hendrickson MR & Kempson RL (1980). Smooth muscle neoplasms. In *Surgical Pathology of the Uterus*, p. 472. Philadelphia: Saunders.

2. Kjerulff KH, Langenberg P, Seidman JD, Stolley PD & Guzinski GM (1996). Uterine leiomyomas: racial differences in severity, symptoms and age at diagnosis. *J Reprod Med* **41**(7): 483–90.

3. Cramer SF & Patel A (1990). The frequency of uterine leiomyomas. *Am J Clin Pathol* **94**: 435–8.

4. Marshall LM, Spiegelman D, Barbieri RL, Goldman MB, Manson JE, Colditz GA, Willett WC & Hunter DJ (1997). Variation in the incidence of uterine leiomyoma among premenopausal women by age and race. *Obstet Gynecol* **90**: 967–73.

5. Baird DD, Schectman JM, Dixon D, Sandler DP & Hill MC (1998). African Americans at higher risk than whites for uterine fibroids: ultrasound evidence (abstract). *Am J Epidemiol* **147**(11): S90.

6. Borgfeldt C & Andolf E (2000). Transvaginal ultrasonographic findings in the uterus and the endometrium: low prevalence of leiomyoma in a random sample of women age 25–40 years. *Acta Obstet Gynecol Scand* **79**: 202–7.

7. Ochai KM, Oda M, Omura M & Tanaka T (2000). Morbidity of uterine fibroids in Japanese women. *Obstet Gynecol* **95**(4): 32S.

8. Velebil P, Wingo PA, Xia Z, Wilcox LS & Peterson HB (1995). Rate of hospitalization for gynecologic disorders among reproductive-age women in the United States. *Obstet Gynecol* **86**: 764–9.

9. Brett KM, Marsh JV & Madans JH (1997). Epidemiology of hysterectomy in the United States: demographic and reproductive factors in a nationally representative sample. *J Women's Health* **6**(3): 309–16.

10. Wilcox LS, Koonin LM, Pokras R, Strauss LT, Xia Z & Peterson, HB (1994). Hysterectomy in the United States, 1988–1990. *Obstet Gynecol* **83**(4): 549–55.

11. Farquhar CM & Steiner CA (2002). Hysterectomy rates in the United States 1990–1997. *Obstet Gynecol* **99**(2): 229–34.

12. Pokras R & Hufnagel VG (1988). Hysterectomy in the United States, 1965–84. *Am J Public Health* **78**: 852–3.

13. Bachmann GA (1990). Hysterectomy: a critical review. *J Reprod Med* **35**(9): 839–862.

14. Allard P & Rochette L (1991). The descriptive epidemiology of hysterectomy, Province of Quebec, 1981–1988. *Ann Epidemiol* **1**: 541–9.

15. Hall RE & Cohen MM (1994). Variations in hysterectomy rates in Ontario: does the indication matter? *Can Med Assoc J* **151**(12): 1713–19.

16. Luoto R, Keskimaki I & Reunanen A (1997). Socioeconomic variations in hysterectomy: evidence from a linkage study of the Finnish hospital discharge register and population census. *J Epidemiol Community Health* **51**: 67–73.

17. Vuorma S, Teperi J, Hurskainen R, Keskimaki I & Kujansuu E (1998). Hysterectomy trends in Finland in 1987–1995. *Acta Obstet Gynecol Scand* **77**: 770–776.

18. Chapron C, Laforest L, Ansquer Y, Fauconnier A, Fernandez B, Breart G & Dubuisson JB (1999). Hysterectomy techniques used for benign pathologies: results of a French multicentre study. *Hum Reprod* **14**(10): 2464–70.

19. Chryssikopoulos A & Loghis C (1986). Indication and results of total hysterectomy. *Int Surg* **71**: 188–94.

20. Gimbel H, Settnes A & Tabor A (2001). Hysterectomy on benign indication in Denmark 1988–1998. *Acta Obstet Gynecol Scand* **80**: 267–72.

21. Vessey MP, Villiard-Mackintosh L, McPherson K, Coulter A & Yeates D (1992). The epidemiology of hysterectomy: findings in a large cohort study. *Br J Obstet Gynaecol* **99**: 402–7.

22. Ross RK, Pike MC, Vessey MP, Bull D, Yeates D & Casagrande JT (1986). Risk factors for uterine fibroids: reduced risk associated with oral contraceptives. *Br Med J* **293**: 359–62.

23. Lumbiganon P, Rugpao S, Phandhu-Fung S, Laopaiboon M, Vudhikamraksa N & Werawatakul Y (1995). Protective effect of depot-medroxyprogesterone acetate on surgically treated uterine leiomyomas: a multicentre case-control study. *Br J Obstet Gynaecol* **103**: 909–14.

24. Faerstein E, Szklo M & Rosenhein N (2001). Risk factors for uterine leiomyoma: a practice-based case-control study. I. African-American heritage, reproductive history, body size, and smoking. *Am J Epidemiol* **153**: 1–10.

25. Parazzini F, Negri E, LaVecchia C, Chatenoud L, Ricci E & Guarnerio P (1996). Reproductive factors and risk of uterine fibroids. *Epidemiology* **7**(4): 440–2.

26. Romieu I, Walker AM & Jick S (1991). Determinants of uterine fibroids. *Post Market Surveil* **5**: 119–33.

27. Chen CR, Buck GM, Courey NG, Perez KM & Wactawski-Wende J (2001). Risk factors for uterine fibroids among women undergoing tubal sterilization. *Am J Epidemiol* **153**: 20–6.

28. Parazzini F, Negri E, La Vecchia C, Fedele L, Rabaiotti M & Luchini L (1992). Oral contraceptive use and risk of uterine fibroids. *Obstet Gynecol* **79**(3): 430–33.

29. Samadi AR, Lee NC, Flanders WD, Boring JR & Parris EB (1996). Risk factors for self-reported uterine fibroids: a case-control study. *Am J Public Health* **86**: 858–62.

30. Meilahn EN, Matthews KA, Egeland G & Kelsey SF (1989). Characteristics of women with hysterectomy. *Maturitas* **11**: 319–29.

31. Balloch EA, (1984). The relative frequency of fibroid processes in the dark-skinned races. *Med News* **1**(xiv): 29.

32. Kjerulff KH, Guzinski GM, Langenberg PW, Stolley PD, Adler Moye NE & Kazandjian VA (1993). Hysterectomy and race. *Obstet Gynecol.* **82**(5): 757–64.

33. Schwartz SM, Marshall LM & Baird DD (2000). Epidemiologic contributions to understanding the etiology of uterine leiomyomata. *Environ Health Perspect* **108**(Suppl 5): 821–7.

33a. Marshall LM, Spiegelman D, Goldman MB, Manson JE, Colditz GA, Barbieri RL, Stampfer MJ & Hunter DJ (1998). A prospective study of reproductive factors and oral contraceptive use in relation to the risk of uterine leiomyomata. *Fertil Steril* **70**(3): 432–9.

34. Sato F, Miyake H, Nishi M & Kudo R (2000). Fertility and uterine size among Asian women undergoing hysterectomy for leiomyomas. *Int J Fertil* **45**(1): 34–7.

35. Rein MS, Barbieri RL & Friedman AJ (1995). Progesterone: a critical role in the pathogenesis of uterine myomas. *Am J Obstet Gynecol* **172**(1): 14–18.

36. Friedman AJ, Hoffman DI, Comite F, Browneller RW & Miller JD (1991). Treatment of leiomyomata uteri with leuprolide acetate depot: a double-blind, placebo-controlled, multicenter study. *Obstet Gynecol* **77**(5): 720–5.

37. Murphy AA, Kettel LM, Morales AJ, Roberts VJ & Yen SS (1993). Regression of uterine leiomyomata in response to the antiprogesterone RU 486. *J Clin Endocrinol Metab* **76**(2): 513–7.

38. Tiltman AJ (1985). The effect of progestins on the mitotic activity of uterine fibroids. *Int J Gynecol Pathol* **4**(2): 89–96.

39. Walker CL, Cesen-Cummings K, Houle C, Baird D, Barrett JC & Davis B (2001). Protective effect of pregnancy for development of uterine leiomyoma. *Carcinogenesis* **22**(12): 2049–52.

40. Ramcharan S, Pellegrin FA, Ray RM & Hsu JP (1980). The Walnut Creek Contraceptive Drug Study. A prospective study of the side effects of oral contraceptives. Vol. III, An interim report: a comparison of disease occurrence leading to hospitalization or death in users and nonusers of oral contraceptives. *J Reprod Med* **25**(Suppl 6): 345–72.

41. Royal College of General Practioners (1974). *Oral Contraceptives and Health.* New York: Pitman Medical Publishing.

42. Schlesselman JJ (1991). Oral contraceptives and neoplasia of the uterine corpus. *Contraception* **43**(6): 557–79.

43. Ratner H (1986). Risk factors for uterine fibroids: reduced risk associated with oral contraceptives. *Br Med J* **293**: 1027.

44. Ikomi AA & Singer A (1997). Protective effect of depot-medroxyprogesterone acetate on surgically treated uterine leiomyomas: a multicentre case-control study. (Letter;comment.) *Br J Obstet Gynaecol* **104**: 385.

45. Bassaw K & Ganger K (1997). Protective effect of depot-medroxyprogesterone acetate on surgically treated uterine leiomyomas:a multicentre case-control study. (Letter; comment.) *Br J Obstet Gynaecol* **104**: 758–9.

46. Frigo P, Eppel W, Asseryanis E, Sator M, Golaszewski T, Gruber D, Lang C & Huber J (1995). The effects of hormone substitution in depot form on the uterus in a group of 50

perimenopausal women – a vaginosonographic study. *Maturitas* **21**: 221–5.

47. Polatti F, Viazzo F, Colleoni R & Nappi RE (2000). Uterine myoma in postmenopause: a comparison between two therapeutic schedules of HRT. *Maturitas* **37**: 27–32.

48. Fedele L, Bianchi S, Raffaelli R & Zanconato G (2000). A randomized study of the effects of tibolone and transdermal estrogen replacement therapy in postmenopausal women with uterine myomas. *Euro J Obstet Gynecol Reprod Bio* **88**: 91–4.

49. Sener AB, Seckin NC, Ozmen S, Gokmen O, Dogu N & Ekici E (1996). The effects of hormone replacement therapy on uterine fibroids in postmenopausal women. *Fertil Steril* **65**(2): 354–7.

50. Ylostalo P, Granberg S, Backstrom AC & Hirsjarvi-Lahti T (1996). Uterine findings by transvaginal sonography during percutaneous estrogen treatment in postmenopausal women. *Maturitas* **23**: 313–17.

51. Colacurci N, De Franciscis P, Cobellis L, Nazzaro G & De Placido G (2000). Effects of hormone replacement therapy on postmenopausal uterine myoma. *Maturitas* **35**: 167–73.

52. Palomba S, Sena T, Noia R, Di Carlo C, Zullo F & Mastrantonio P (2001). Transdermal hormone replacement therapy in postmenopausal women with uterine leiomyomas. *Obstet Gynecol* **98**(6): 1053–8.

53. De Aloysio D, Altieri P, Penacchioni P, Salgarello M & Ventura V (1998). Bleeding patterns in recent postmenopausal outpatients with uterine myomas: comparison between two regimens of HRT. *Maturitas* **29**: 261–4.

54. Gregoriou O, Vitoratos N, Papadias C, Konidaris S, Costomenos D & Chryssikopoulos A (1997). Effect of tibolone on postmenopausal women with myomas. *Maturitas* **27**: 187–91.

55. Palomba S, Sammartino A, Di Carlo C, Affinito P, Zullo F & Nappi C (2001). Effects of raloxifene treatment on uterine leiomyomas in postmenopausal women. *Fertil Steril* **76**(1): 38–43.

56. Wahab M, Thompson J & Al-Azzawi F (2000). The effect of submucous fibroids on the dose-dependent modulation of uterine bleeding by trimegestone in postmenopausal women treated with hormone replacement therapy. *Br J Obstet Gynaecol* **107**: 329–34.

57. Townsend DE, Fields G, McCausland A & Kauffman K (1993). Diagnostic and operative hysteroscopy in the management of persistent postmenopausal bleeding. *Obstet Gynecol* **82**(3): 419–21.

58. Andersen J & Barbieri RL (1995). Abnormal gene expression in uterine leiomyomas. *J Soc Gynecol Invest* **2**: 663–72.

59. Marshall LM, Speigelman D, Manson JE, Goldman MB, Barbieri RL, Stampfer MJ, Willett WC & Hunter DJ (1998). Risk of uterine leiomyomata among premenopausal women in relation to body size and cigarette smoking. *Epidemiology* **9**(5): 511–17.

60. Okoronkwo MO (1999). Body weight and uterine leiomyomas among women in Nigeria. *West African J Med* **18**(1): 52–4.

61. Sato F, Nishi M, Kudo R & Miyake H (1998). Body fat distribution and uterine leiomyomas. *J Epidemiol* **8**: 176–80.

62. Baron JA, La Vecchia C & Levi F (1990). The antiestrogenic effect of cigarette smoking in women. *Am J Obstet Gynecol* **162**: 502–14.

63. Parazzini F, Negri F, La Vecchia C, Rabaiotti M, Luchini L, Villa A & Fedele L (1996). Uterine myomas and smoking. Results from an Italian study. *J Reprod Med* **41**(5): 316–20.

64. Chiaffarino F, Parazzini F, La Vecchia C, Chatenoud L, Di Cintio E & Marsico S (1999). Diet and uterine myomas. *Obstet Gynecol* **94**(3): 395–8.

65. Wyshak G, Frisch RE, Albright NL, Albright TE & Schiff I (1986). Lower prevalence of benign diseases of the breast and benign tumours of the reproductive system among former college athletes compared to non-athletes. *Br J Cancer* **54**: 841–5.

66. Schwartz SM (2001). Epidemiology of uterine leiomyomata. *Clin Obstet Gynecol* **44**(2): 316–32.

66a. Parazzini F, La Vecchia C, Negri E, Cecchetti GS Fedele L (1988). Epidemiologic characteristics of women with uterine fibroids: a case-control study. *Obstet Gynecol* **72**(6): 853–7.

67. Faerstein E, Szklo M & Rosenshein NB (2001). Risk factors for uterine leiomyoma: A practice-based case-control study. II. Atherogenic risk factors and potential sources of uterine irritation. *Am J Epidemiol* **153**(1): 11–19.

68. Luoto R, Rutanen EM & Auvinen A (2001). Fibroids and hypertension. A cross-sectional study of women undergoing hysterectomy. *J Reprod Med* **46**(4): 359–64.

69. Kurbanova M, Koroleva AG & Sergeev AS (1989). Genetic-epidemiological analysis of uterine myoma: estimate of risk to relatives. *Genetika* **25**: 1896–8.

70. Vikhlyaeva EM, Khodzhaeva ZS & Fantschenko ND (1995). Familial predisposition to uterine leiomyomas. *Int J Gynecol Obstet* **51**: 127–31.

71. Luoto R, Kaprio J, Rutanen EM, Taipale P, Perola M & Koskenvuo M (2000). Heritability and risk factors of uterine fibroids – the Finnish twin cohort-study. *Maturitas* **37**: 15–26.

72. Ligon AH & Morton CC (2001). Leiomyomata: heritability and cytogenic studies. *Hum Reprod Update* **7**(1): 8–14.

73. Van de Ven WJ (1998). Genetic basis of uterine leiomyoma: involvement of high mobility group protein genes. *Europ J Obstet Gynecol Reprod Bio* **81**: 289–93.

2

Histopathology of uterine leiomyomas

Charles V. Biscotti and Tommaso Falcone

Cleveland Clinic Foundation, Ohio, USA

Uterine leiomyomas are monoclonal smooth muscle tumors.[1-3] Early research on isoform analysis of glucose-6-phosphate dehydrogenase in the smooth muscle cells of uterine leiomyomas pointed to the monoclonal nature of this tumor. Each leiomyoma lesion in the uterus may have a distinct isoform and are presumed to arise independently. Cytogenetic abnormalities of several chromosomes have been identified within these smooth muscle tumors with normal karyotype in the adjacent non-tumorous regions. These cytogenetic mutations have been identified in about 40% of uterine leiomyomas. Some of the mutations involve genes involved in cellular growth regulation.[4,5] Correlation between the genotype of the leiomyomas and the phenotype has not led to conclusive observations.

Gross morphology

Uterine leiomyomas are usually well-circumscribed tumors. They can occur in any part of the uterus, including the cervix. They may also occur in the round ligaments. Generally they are divided into subserosal, intramural, and submucosal. The subserosal and submucosal uterine leiomyomas can become pedunculated. The submucosal uterine leiomyomas can protrude into the uterine cavity or become pedunculated, and protrude through the cervix. Uterine leiomyomas can become separated from the uterus, and can be found in different areas such as the retroperitoneal space between the leaves of the broad ligament of the uterus.

These parasitic uterine leiomyomas derive their blood supply from other sources such as omental vessels.

On section, these tumors distort the myometrium or the uterine cavity. They are composed of whorled rubbery firm pink–white bulging tissue and they have no true capsule. Myoma can be calcified, cystic, or degenerated.

On gross examination, an adenomyoma or localized adenomyosis may be confused with a leiomyoma. A cleavage plane seen in myoma is not found in adenomyoma. As a result, excision of an adenomyoma is difficult. The diagnosis of adenomyoma or adenomyosis can be made histopathologically, by magnetic resonance imaging (MRI) and occasionally by ultrasound.

Degeneration of leiomyoma can occur through several mechanisms. Interruption of its blood supply causes necrosis and gives a yellowish appearance. Hemorrhage inside the myoma is seen as a dark hemorrhagic central area. Red or carneous degeneration occurs after a more acute interruption of the blood supply such as during pregnancy or after uterine embolization. Hyaline degeneration refers to the extensive deposition of collagen to the extent of replacing all the smooth muscle. Calcification can occur after extensive degeneration.

Histopathology of a typical leiomyoma

The typical uterine leiomyoma consists of smooth muscle cells with elongated, uniform nuclei. The smooth muscle cells are arranged in interlacing bundles. Mitotic figures are inconspicuous, usually fewer than one per 10 high magnification fields. By definition, mitotic activity is less than five mitotic figures per 10 high magnification fields.

Histopathology of an atypical leiomyoma

The most common atypical histologic variants include those with increased cellularity (cellular leiomyomas) and those with increased mitotic activity (mitotically active leiomyomas). Cellular leiomyomas have closely packed spindle shaped nuclei creating a densely cellular appearance. However, other worrisome histologic features are lacking. A report to the gynecologist of a cellular leiomyoma is not worrisome.

Cellular leiomyomas can be confused histologically with endometrial stromal neoplasms. However, variably sized blood vessels including thick-walled blood vessels, a conspicuous fascicular pattern, merging with the adjacent myometrium, and the absence of stromal foam cells favor the diagnosis of leiomyoma and argue against a stromal neoplasm.

Other histologic variants of leiomyoma include bizarre leiomyoma, hemorrhagic/apoplectic leiomyoma, epithelioid leiomyoma, myxoid leiomyoma, vascular leiomyoma, lipoleiomyoma, diffuse leiomyomatosis, intravenous leiomyomatosis and hydropic degeneration. Bizarre leiomyomas are characterized by marked nuclear atypia characterized by bizarre giant nuclei and multinucleated giant cells. These leiomyomas lack other histologic features of malignancy. Specifically, mitotic activity is low, almost always less than five mitotic figures per 10 high power fields and tumor cell necrosis is lacking. Also, the gross appearance of bizarre leiomyomas does not deviate from the usual leiomyoma.

Hemorrhagic or apoplectic leiomyomas have patchy areas of hemorrhage, often associated with a slight increase in mitotic activity. Other worrisome histologic features are lacking. Polygonal tumor cells

characterize epithelioid leiomyomas rather than the usual elongate spindle shaped tumor cells. Myxoid leiomyomas have abundant extracellular mucin. Myxoid leiomyomas are extremely uncommon and the presence of myxoid change should raise the possibility of a myxoid leiomyosarcoma. Myxoid leiomyomas are sharply circumscribed tumors unlike myxoid leiomyosarcomas, which characteristically have an infiltrative margin.

Vascular leiomyomas contain numerous variably sized blood vessels but otherwise resemble typical leiomyomas. Lipoleiomyomas contain benign adipose tissue. Diffuse leiomyomatosis has innumerable smooth muscle nodules throughout the myometrium. Intravenous leiomyomatosis has benign smooth muscle nodules growing within veins. The smooth muscle nodules resemble typical leiomyomas; however, the lesions of intravenous leiomyomatosis often have more prominent vasculature. Leiomyomas with hydropic degeneration have abundant extracellular edema. Unlike myxoid leiomyomas, the extracellular edema stains negatively with mucin stains.

Histopathology of leiomyosarcomata

These tumors appear gross as soft, variegated masses with hemorrhage and necrosis. Histologically, the three key diagnostic features include nuclear atypia, increased mitotic activity, and tumor cell necrosis. Mitoses are usually numerous and easily identified, exceeding 10 mitotic figures per high power field in the vast majority of tumors.

Effect of gonadotropin-releasing hormone (GnRH) agonists

Reports of the histopathology of leiomyomas after treatment with GnRH agonists have been contradictory.[6] Increased, decreased, and no change in cellularity of the surgically removed leiomyoma have all been reported. Hyaline degeneration of the excised

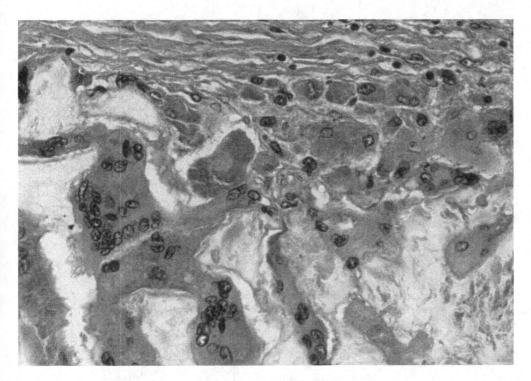

Figure 2.1. Post-embolization specimens characteristically have intravascular foreign body giant cell reaction in peripheral blood vessels. (Hematoxylin and eosin, original magnification × 62.2.) See also color plates.

leiomyoma has been observed. It is associated with a decreased vessel lumen size that is presumably the result of hypoestrogenemia with a resulting ischemia.

Histopathology of the post-embolization leiomyoma

There is very little data of the histopathology of the uterus after uterine artery embolization. The few case reports are from uteri that have been removed as a result of a complication after embolization and may not be representative of all cases.[7,8] There are several post-embolization clinical situations that will require surgery. These include prolapse of a fibroid through the cervix, expulsion of tissue through the cervix, sepsis, persistent symptoms of pain, and bleeding.

In 10 patients who passed the myoma spontaneously through the vagina and who underwent a hysterectomy after embolization, the primary features of the myoma were thrombosis and necrosis. Several weeks after embolization, there was extensive coagulative necrosis and acute inflammation. Months after the procedure the primary features were of hyaline necrosis and dystrophic calcification.

In a patient with a leiomyosarcoma, large areas of hyaline necrosis were seen. Foreign materials are almost always found within the blood vessels representing the polyvinyl alcohol used for embolization. These foreign materials are surrounded by a histiocytic and giant cell reaction.

Myoma after embolization shows gross and microscopic features of an infarcted leiomyoma. The findings vary with the interval between embolization and excision. In general, the specimens have well developed coagulation necrosis. Grossly, the

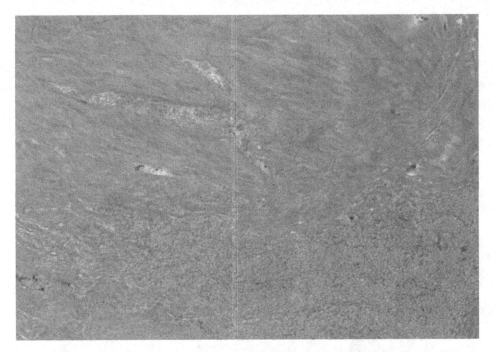

Figure 2.2. This post-embolization myoma has well developed coagulation necrosis characterized by loss of nuclei (karyolysis) and eosinophilia (top of field) and a hemorrhagic zone (bottom). (Hematoxylin and eosin, original magnification × 62.2.) See also color plates.

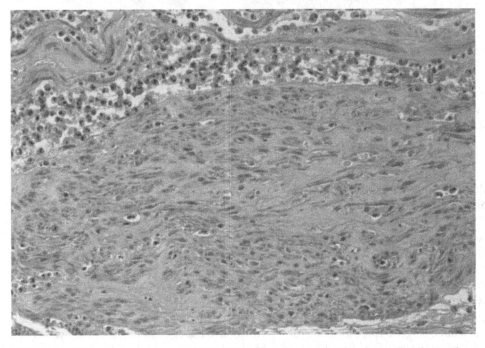

Figure 2.3. Neutrophils infiltrate from the periphery of this infarcted leiomyoma. Necrotic myofibers have well developed coagulation necrosis with cytoplasmic eosinophilia and loss of nuclei (karyolysis). (Hematoxylin and eosin, original magnification × 62.2.) See also color plates.

myomas have a dusky red softening in contrast to the characteristic firm, white whorled appearance of a myoma. Histologically, foreign body emboli can be seen in blood vessels at the periphery (Figure 2.1, see also color plates). Another finding is coagulation necrosis that is characterized by cytoplasmic eosinophilia and loss of (karyolysis) or fragmentation of (karyorrhexis) nuclei (Figure 2.2, see also color plates).

Case presentation 1

A 50-year-old woman with persistent symptoms of menorrhagia underwent a supracervical hysterectomy four months after uterine artery embolization. The pathology showed leiomyoma and an intravascular giant cell reaction to foreign material and an endometritis. (Figure 2.1, see also color plates).

Case presentation 2

One year and four months after uterine artery embolization, a 46-year-old woman underwent a hysterectomy. A necrotic leiomyoma was found. (See Figure 2.2 and color plates.)

Case presentation 3

Due to persistent bleeding, a 40-year-old woman underwent a hysterectomy three weeks after uterine artery embolization. (See Figure 2.3 and color plates.)

REFERENCES

1. Benda J (2001). Pathology of smooth muscle tumors of the uterine corpus. *Clin Obstet Gynecol* **44**: 350–63.
2. Crow J (1998). Pathology of uterine fibroids. *Balliere's Clin Obstet Gynecol* **12**: 197–211.
3. Wilkinson N & Rollason TP (2001). Recent advances in the pathology of smooth muscle tumors of the uterus. *Histopathology* **39**: 331–41.
4. Gross KL & Morton CC (2001). Genetics and the development of fibroids. *Clin Obstet Gynecol* **44**: 335–49.
5. Layfield LJ, Liu K, Dodge R & Barsky SH (2000). Uterine smooth muscle tumors: utility of classification by proliferation, ploidy, and prognostic markers versus traditional histopathology. *Arch Pathol Lab Med* **124**: 221–7.
6. Sreenan JJ, Prayson RA & Biscotti CV et al. (1996). Histopathologic findings in 107 uterine leiomyomas treated with leuprolide acetate compared with 126 controls. *Am J Surg Pathol* **20**: 427–32.
7. McCluggage WG, Ellis PK, McClure N, Walker WJ, Jackson PA & Manek S (2000). Pathologic features of uterine leiomyomas following uterine artery embolization. *Int J Gynecol Pathol* **19**: 342–7.
8. Nicholson TA, Pelage JP & Ettles DF (2001). Fibroid calcification after uterine artery embolization: ultrasonographic appearance and pathology. *J Vasc Interv Radiol* **12**: 443–6.

3

Imaging of uterine leiomyomas

Giovanni Artho,[1] Caroline Reinhold,[1,2] and Ida Khalili[1]

[1] McGill University Health Center, Quebec, Canada
[2] Synarc Inc., California, USA

Role of imaging

The role of imaging is to confirm the diagnosis of uterine leiomyoma and to differentiate leiomyomas from other causes of uterine enlargement or pelvic masses such as ovarian or endometrial based masses, adenomyosis, serosal implants and lymphadenopathy. In addition, the number, size, and location of leiomyomas must be assessed. This is particularly important in the symptomatic, infertile, or pregnant patient. Possible complications including benign degeneration should be recognized. Signs suggestive of malignant transformation must be evaluated. Imaging is useful in preoperative mapping, particularly in the setting of uterus-sparing procedures and for therapy monitoring.

General histology

Uterine leiomyomas are well-circumscribed, benign smooth muscle neoplasms with various amounts of fibrous connective tissue. Leiomyomas may be single or, more frequently, multiple.[1] Uterine leiomyomata are estrogen-sensitive neoplasms that occur in 20–30% of reproductive-aged women. Leiomyomas regress during anovulatory cycles as a result of unopposed estrogen stimulation. As leiomyomas enlarge, they may outgrow their blood supply, resulting in ischemia and degeneration characterized as hyaline, cystic, myxomatous, fatty, or hemorrhagic.[2] Rapid increase in size of leiomyomas in a post-menopausal patient should raise the possibility of sarcomatous change.

Classification by location

Leiomyomas originate from the uterine corpus in the vast majority of cases; however, rarely (3–8%) they can arise from the cervical region.[2,3] Uterine leiomyomas are categorized with respect to their location (subserosal, intramural, submucosal). This classification is of clinical significance because the symptoms and treatment vary among these different subtypes (Figure 3.1):[1]

- *Subserosal* leiomyomas occur when more than 50% of the volume extends outside the uterine contours. Occasionally, a fibroid will be seen as a mass in the right adnexa or broad ligament (pedunculated or intraligamentary).
- *Intramural* leiomyomas are located within the myometrium.
- *Submucosal* leiomyomas occur when more than 50% of the volume protrudes into the endometrial cavity.

Imaging modalities

Plain radiography

Plain radiography has no role in the evaluation of leiomyomas. Non-specific changes such as mass effect on adjacent bowel and urinary bladder, as well as increased density of the pelvis may be seen with large and multiple leiomyomas. Leiomyomas are not directly visualized on plain radiographs unless the tumor has undergone calcification, which typically appear as coarse and irregular. This type of change is most common with pedunculated subserosal tumors, and in leiomyomas occurring in postmenopausal women.

During intravenous pyelography, leiomyomas may be detected as non-specific pelvic masses compressing the ureters and causing hydronephrosis.

Ultrasound

Technique
Ultrasound (US) is the ideal modality to confirm the clinically suspected diagnosis. US provides adequate answers to the vast majority of clinical questions. It is useful in the diagnosis of uterine leiomyomas and differentiating this condition from other gynecological pathology. However, US at times is suboptimal for accurately defining the location of uterine leiomyomas.[4] An additional limitation of US is its operator dependence.

Transabdominal ultrasound (TAS) is technically the simplest and fastest examination. Probes for TAS generally use frequencies on the order of 3 to 5 MHz, which provide the necessary penetration for imaging organs posterior to the urinary bladder but suffer from limited spatial resolution. TAS is ideal for overall assessment of an enlarged uterus, particularly in the presence of large, multiple, and/or markedly calcified fibroids. In our experience, the resolution afforded by TAS is not sufficient to demonstrate the more subtle leiomyomas, to differentiate leiomyomas from adenomyosis, and to accurately localize the leiomyomas. *Endovaginal ultrasound (EVS)* offers several advantages over TAS. There is better depiction of the uterine anatomy through placement of the transducer in the vaginal vault and avoidance of subcutaneous fat.[5] EVS allows the use of higher-frequency transducers, improving the spatial resolution[3] and reducing imaging artefacts.[6] A disadvantage is the limited field of view particularly in retroverted or enlarged myomatous uteri, where the fundus may be located beyond the focal zone of

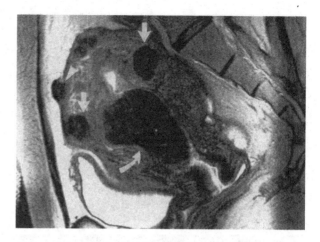

Figure 3.1. Classification by location. Sagittal T2-weighted MR image of the uterus demonstrates multiple, non-degenerated leiomyomas in submucosal (curved arrow), intramural (arrows) and subserosal (arrowhead) locations. (Reprinted with permission from Wiley-Liss, New York. See Ref. 15.)

the transducer. In addition, large pedunculated fibroids may go undetected. Hence, the endovaginal approach should be used in conjunction with TAS.

Hysterosonography is performed in conjunction with EVS and involves the instillation of sterile saline into the endometrial cavity to promote distension. Hysterosonography is highly accurate at: (1) classifying a leiomyoma as submucosal in location (Figure 3.2); and (2) differentiating it from endometrial-based masses such as endometrial polyps or cancer. To prepare the patient for a hysterosonogram, a sterile speculum is inserted and the cervix is cleansed with an antiseptic solution. A catheter, usually a hysterosalpingography catheter is inserted into the uterine cavity. A water-filled balloon prevents the retrograde leakage of saline into the vagina.

Imaging findings
On ultrasound, the uterus may be enlarged and heterogeneous with a globular contour due to multiple, small leiomyomas. Focal leiomyomas have a variable sonographic appearance. The most common sonographic appearance is a round, whorled, and well defined mass (Figure 3.3). Depending on its size and

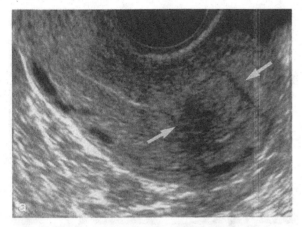

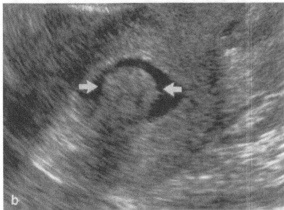

Figure 3.2. Endovaginal ultrasound (EVS) appearance and hysterosonography. (a) Sagittal EVS in a patient with a retroverted uterus shows a hypoechoic, whorled, attenuating mass (arrows) consistent with a leiomyoma. The exact location of the leiomyoma, submucosal versus mural is uncertain. (b) Transverse section of the uterus after hysterosonography confirms the myometrial origin of the mass (arrows), and furthermore, establishes the submucosal location of the leiomyoma.

location, resultant deformity of the external uterine contour or distortion of the endometrial lining is frequent. The echotexture depends on the relative ratio of fibrous tissue to smooth muscle and on the presence and type of degeneration.[2] Hence, leiomyomas are variable in appearance, however most commonly present as hypoechoic and heterogeneous masses (Figures 3.2 and 3.3). Echogenic areas may be

seen with calcific, hemorrhagic or fatty degeneration (Figure 3.4). Anechoic areas are seen in leiomyomas with cystic degeneration.[2] Acoustic attenuation or shadowing is commonly encountered with calcific degeneration in association with a bright focus (Figure 3.3a). However, leiomyomas without calcification frequently demonstrate edge shadowing and some degree of sound attenuation. A pseudocapsule of compressed areolar tissue containing one or two feeding vessels is frequently seen surrounding the tumor. These peripheral vessels can be seen with color Doppler interrogation (Figure 3.5, see also color plates). Measurements of peak systolic velocity or impedance of the uterine and intralesional vessels are not specific, and can be used neither to diagnose leiomyomas nor to differentiate them from other pathologic conditions with any degree of confidence.

Differential diagnosis
The group of differential diagnoses to be considered will depend largely on the location of the leiomyoma in question. For myometrial-based leiomyomas, differentiation from *adenomyosis* pre-operatively is essential, since uterine-conserving therapy is possible with leiomyomas whereas hysterectomy is the definitive treatment for debilitating adenomyosis.[6] EVS represents a substantial improvement over transabdominal ultrasound to reliably differentiate these two common myometrial lesions. On EVS, adenomyosis typically presents as poorly defined, heterogeneous areas of decreased myometrial echogenicity with or without small myometrial cysts (Figure 3.6).[7] In contradistinction to leiomyomas, adenomyosis has minimal or no mass effect on surrounding structures and tends to maintain an elliptical shape along the long-axis of the uterus.[8] An exception is the adenomyoma, which can mimic a leiomyoma in every respect. Color Doppler interrogation of fibroids frequently demonstrates a rim of peripherally located feeding vessels; whereas in adenomyosis, a diffuse speckled pattern of moderate color Doppler flow within the lesion is common. *Myometrial contractions* may also mimic leiomyomas. Myometrial contractions typically evolve during the course of the US examination and thus

are recognized by their changing or vanishing behavior. Submucosal leiomyomas need to be differentiated from endometrial pathology, such as
polyps or cancer. A round, hypoechoic, well delineated mass, bridging myo- and endometrium
characterizes a submucosal fibroid. Endometrial
polyps present as a focal or diffuse thickening of
the endometrium and are most often hyperechoic.
Larger polyps frequently have small areas of cystic
change. The presence of stalk flow on color Doppler,
favors the diagnosis of an endometrial polyp, but
is not entirely specific. In patients where the differentiation of an endometrial-based mass versus a
submucosal leiomyoma remains unclear, hysterosonography is often a definitive test. The differential diagnosis of a subserosal or intraligamentary
fibroid includes *ovarian pathology*, for example ovarian fibroma/fibrothecoma, endometrioma, or primary and secondary solid ovarian neoplasms. In the
absence of a separately identified, normal-appearing
ovary on the ipsilateral side, differentiating pedunculated leiomyomas from ovarian pathology is
difficult on ultrasound, and these patients benefit
from further evaluation with magnetic resonance
imaging (MRI). The diagnosis of *leiomyosarcoma* is
made in the setting of a myometrial-based mass with:
(1) a history of rapid growth (particularly worrisome in the postmenopausal patient); (2) irregular
or ill-defined borders; or (3) evidence of local or
distant spread. The echotexture or homogeneity of
the lesion, as well as Doppler indices, are of no
value in differentiating leiomyomas from leiomyosarcomas.

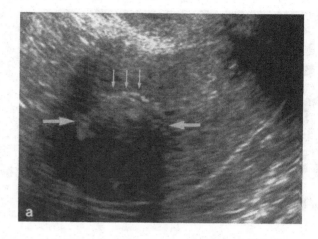

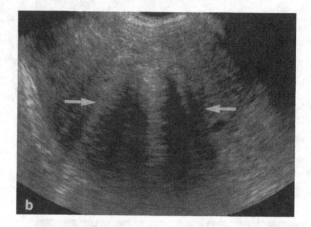

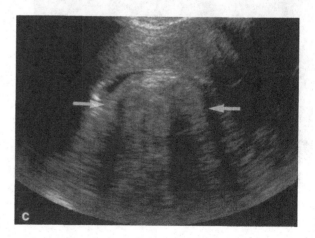

Figure 3.3. Endovaginal ultrasound (EVS) appearance and
hysterosonography. (a) Sagittal and (b, c) transverse EVS
sections in two different patients demonstrate well-defined,
round, hypoechoic masses (arrows) with a whorled
appearance and areas of attenuation. Calcifications (small
arrows) (a) are present along the anterior border of this mural
leiomyoma, which displaces the endometrial lining ventrally.
The exact location of the leiomyoma in the second patient
(b) is uncertain from EVS alone. Hysterosonography (c), by
outlining the endometrial lining confirms the mural location
of the leiomyoma.

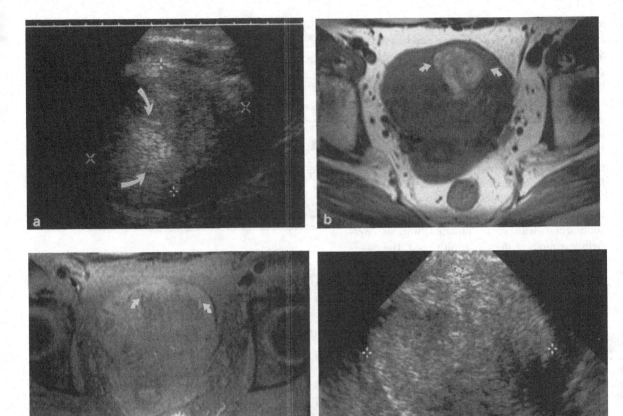

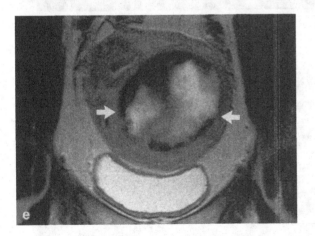

Figure 3.4. Fatty and hemorrhagic degeneration.
(a) Endovaginal ultrasound (EVS) demonstrates a large mass
(calipers) of mixed echogenicity arising from the uterus. Note
the presence of a hyperechoic area (curved arrows) in the
ventral aspect of the mass near the fundus. T1-weighted
transverse sections on magnetic resonance imaging (MRI)
(b) without and (c) with fat suppression in the same patient
confirm the presence of fatty degeneration (curved arrows) of
the leiomyoma. (d) Transverse EVS and (e) coronal
T2-weighted MRI in a different patient illustrate the presence
of red degeneration in a mural leiomyoma (calipers d,
arrows e). Although, the EVS findings are non-specific, the
findings on the T2-weighted MR images are suggestive.
Confirmation was obtained with T1-weighted MR images (not
shown), which showed diffuse hyperintensity indicating the
presence of blood products. (Figure 3.4(b,c,e) Reprinted with
permission from Wiley-Liss, New York. See Ref. 15.)

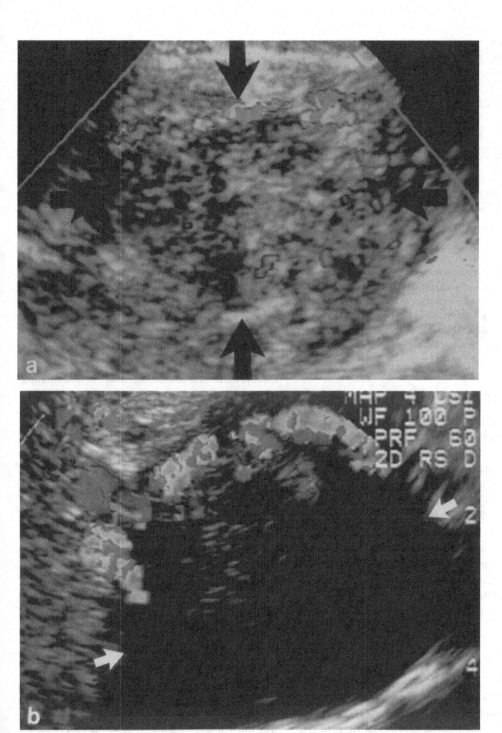

Figure 3.5. Rim of color Doppler. (a) Intramural and (b) subserosal leiomyomas (arrows) in two different patients demonstrate the typical rim of color Doppler flow with endovaginal ultrasound. See also color plates.

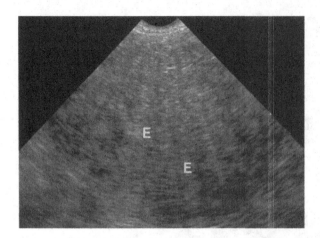

Figure 3.6. Diffuse adenomyosis. Transverse-oblique section through the uterus with endovaginal ultrasound (EVS) in a patient with diffuse adenomyosis demonstrates the myometrium to be hypoechoic and heterogeneous. No mass as such can be identified. Note the poor visualization of the endometrium (E), a frequent finding on EVS in patients with diffuse adenomyosis.

Computed tomography (CT)

CT scanning has no primary role in the evaluation of patients with suspected uterine leiomyomas. This is because of its relatively limited contrast resolution and its reliance on ionizing radiation. On CT scanning, leiomyomas present as solid masses of uniform or slightly heterogeneous consistency in a distorted and/or enlarged uterus. Coarse, dystrophic calcifications are the most specific sign of a leiomyoma. Hyper- and hypovascularity can be seen after intravenous contrast administration. Necrotic areas containing fluid and air can be present within a leiomyoma after uterine artery embolization (UAE), and should not be mistaken for infection.

MRI

Role of MRI

The excellent soft tissue differentiation of MRI makes it an ideal tool for gynecologic imaging as it provides high-contrast, multiplanar and global views of the female pelvis.[5,6] Compared to EVS, MRI is consider-ably less operator-dependant and provides images that are standard and reproducible over time. The high cost and limited availability of MRI, however, makes it an impractical tool for the initial evaluation of patients with suspected leiomyomas. The role of MRI is that of a problem solving modality, in cases where the findings at sonography are inconclusive or technically limited. When used in this way, MRI may obviate the need for surgery or enable more directed and less invasive surgical procedures.[9]

MRI has greater sensitivity for preoperative localization of uterine leiomyomas than does EVS or hysterosonography.[4] Conditions that mimic leiomyomas at physical examination and EVS are usually accurately characterized with MRI.[10] For example, MRI more readily determines the ovarian versus uterine nature of an adnexal mass, whereas US may be non-specific.[10] Adenomyosis can be accurately diagnosed with MRI and differentiated from leiomyomas, while the findings at US may be indeterminate.[11,12] Direct visualization of leiomyomas with respect to the uterine zonal anatomy is important in determining whether sufficient myometrium will remain after myomectomy so that childbearing function can be preserved.[13]

In addition, MRI can differentiate cellular leiomyomas from other histologic subtypes. Since cellular leiomyomas respond better to non-surgical treatment (gonadotropin-releasing hormone, GnRH, analogs or uterine artery embolization), MRI can be used to predict response to medical therapy and potentially select appropriate patients for uterine artery embolization. MRI can be used to monitor, in a standard and reproducible fashion, the results of medical therapy, i.e. GnRH analogs, or uterine artery embolization[1] by demonstrating the degree of volume shrinkage and loss of enhancement of leiomyomas.[14] MRI can also demonstrate post procedural complications such as hematoma, abscess, fistula, uterine rupture, and peritoneal inclusion cyst formation.[1]

Imaging findings – normal uterus

The normal uterine zonal anatomy is best depicted using sagittal T2-weighted sequences. In women of

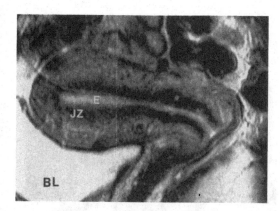

Figure 3.7. Normal uterus on magnetic resonance imaging. Sagittal section through the uterus on a T2-weighted image demonstrates three distinct zones in reproductive age women. The central, high signal intensity stripe represents the normal endometrium (E). Immediately subjacent is a band of low signal intensity referred to as the junctional zone (JZ). This represents the inner myometrium. The outer myometrium is of intermediate signal intensity on T2-weighted images. BL: Urinary bladder.

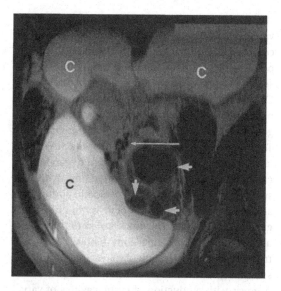

Figure 3.8. Establishing the myometrial origin. Coronal T2-weighted magnetic resonance imaging (MRI) in a patient with a large subserosal leiomyoma demonstrates areas of peripheral cystic (C) degeneration. Feeding vessels (long arrow) originating from the myometrium confirm the myometrial origin of this pedunculated mass. Small, nondegenerated leiomyomas (arrows) can be seen in the body of the uterus. (Reprinted with permission from Wiley-Liss, New York. See Ref. 15.)

reproductive age, three distinct layers are recognized on T2 weighted images (Figure 3.7):

(1) The central, high signal intensity stripe represents the normal endometrium.

(2) Immediately subjacent is a band of low signal intensity referred to as the junctional zone. This is the inner myometrium and is both functionally and structurally different from the outer myometrium. The normal junctional zone has low signal intensity on T2-weighted images.[15] This low signal is hypothesized to be due to the more compact arrangement, and decreased water content of the smooth muscle fibres in the inner myometrium.[16] The junctional zone varies considerably in measurement, with a mean thickness of 2–8mm. The junctional zone is wider and anatomically does not correspond to the subendometrial halo on EVS.

(3) The outer myometrium is of intermediate signal intensity on T2-weighted images. Vascular structures are seen more commonly in the outer myometrium.

Imaging findings – leiomyomas

The diagnosis of a leiomyoma on MRI is made primarily on the basis of its location and morphologic characteristics. The goal is to establish the myometrial origin of the mass, since this significantly limits the differential diagnosis. For pedunculated, subserosal leiomyomas, feeding vessels originating from the myometrium can be taken as presumptive evidence of a myometrial-based mass (Figure 3.8). Signal-intensity characteristics alone are not useful in differentiating leiomyomas from other pathologic conditions, due to the variable appearance of uterine leiomyomas.

The typical MRI appearance of a *non-degenerated leiomyoma* is a well-circumscribed mass of homogeneously decreased signal intensity compared to the outer myometrium on T2-weighted images (Figure 3.1). In addition, leiomyomas are frequently surrounded by a high-intensity rim resulting from vascular congestion.[1,2] A mass is considered an uncomplicated leiomyoma if it is isointense or hypointense to normal myometrium on all pulse sequences and if its margins are well defined.[17] Cellular leiomyomas, which are composed of compact smooth muscle cells, with little or no collagen, can have relatively high signal intensity on T2-weighted images.[1] When a myoma becomes large, oxygen deprivation will lead to degenerative changes. In the early stage of degeneration, hydropic swelling occurs and if impaired blood supply persists, hyaline degeneration, necrosis, and fatty degeneration will occur. *Hyaline degeneration* involves accumulation of proteinaceous tissue in the extra cellular space.[1] Hyaline tissue is an amorphous substance, which has a tendency for liquefactive necrosis with production of cystic cavities of varying size.[18] It is the most frequent type, accounting for 63% of degenerated leiomyomas.[19] Hyaline degenerated myomas have low signal intensity on T2-weighted images, similar to standard leiomyomas. *Cystic degeneration* results in areas of high signal intensity on T2-weighted images, and the cystic areas do not enhance (Figures 3.8 and 3.9).[1] Necrotic leiomyomas that have not liquefied (i.e. *hyaline, coagulative*) have low T2 and variable T1 signal intensities. *Calcification* follows necrosis, and typically presents as areas of signal void on all sequences. *Myxoid degeneration* involves the presence of gelatinous hyaluronic acid-rich mucopolysaccharides.[1] *Myxoid degeneration* results in areas with very high signal intensity on T2-weighted images that demonstrate mild enhancement after gadolinium administration.[1] *Red degeneration* is an infrequent hemorrhagic infarction of leiomyomas occurring most commonly during pregnancy.[20] Red degeneration is considered the result of venous obstruction[20] and may exhibit an unusual signal intensity pattern (Figure 3.4e). On T1-weighted sequences, hemorrhagic infarction typically demonstrates peripheral or diffuse hyperintensity secondary to the presence of blood products. On T2-weighted sequences, the signal is variable with or without a hypointense rim.

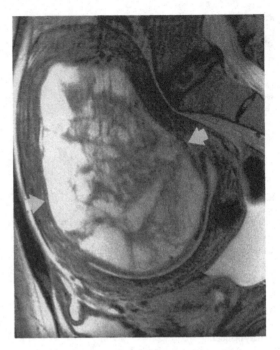

Figure 3.9. Cystic Degeneration. Sagittal T2-weighted magnetic resonance image shows a large leiomyoma arising from the ventral myometrium (arrows). The areas of high signal within represent cystic degeneration. (Reprinted with permission from Wiley-Liss, New York. See Ref. 15.)

The latter is best explained by the presence of intracellular methemoglobin within red blood cells confined to the thrombosed blood vessels surrounding the tumor.[19] Causes for hyperintense signal on T1-weighted images include fatty, cystic, or red degeneration.[20] Rarely, lipomatous uterine tumors, such as lipoleiomyoma or lipoma may also be included in the differential diagnosis (Figures 3.4b and 3.4c).

Differential diagnosis

A *focal myometrial contraction* can appear as a low signal intensity mass on T2-weighted sequences and thus can mimic a leiomyoma or focal adenomyosis.[1,16] The low signal is generated by the more compact smooth muscle cells and compressed venous structures. Resolution or change in the shape of the lesion on follow-up sequences confirms the transient nature and allows the diagnosis to be established.[1] *Adenomyosis* is most commonly a diffuse abnormality but may occur as a focal mass called adenomyoma.[18] The diffuse form appears on MRI as thickening of the junctional zone (>12 mm) with foci of high signal on T2-weighted sequences in 50–88% of cases (Figure 3.10a).[7,21] MRI is highly accurate in diagnosing diffuse adenomyosis and differentiating it from leiomyomas.[7,22] The differentiation of a leiomyoma from an adenomyoma, however, poses a greater challenge. Typically, adenomyomas tend to be less well defined, produce little mass effect and may have an elliptical shape (Figure 3.10b and 3.10c). MRI is highly accurate in differentiating submucosal leiomyomas from *endometrial polyps* by establishing the myometrial origin of the mass. In addition, on T2-weighted sequences small submucosal leiomyomas are usually markedly hypointense, whereas small endometrial polyps tend to be isointense or only mildly hypointense relative to the surrounding endometrium (Figure 3.11).[23] However, larger leiomyomas and polyps are of variable signal intensity on MRI. MRI is superior to EVS in determining the origin of an *adnexal mass*,

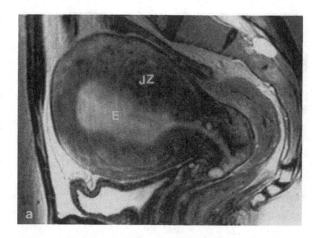

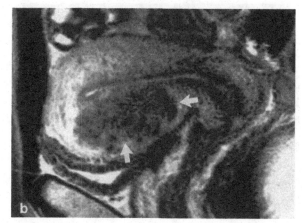

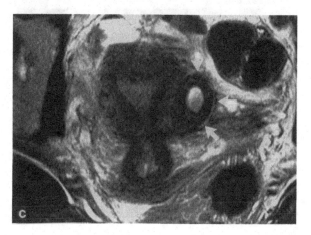

Figure 3.10. Adenomyosis. (a) Sagittal T2-weighted magnetic resonance imaging (MRI) in a patient with diffuse adenomyosis demonstrates thickening of the junctional zone (JZ), more pronounced dorsally. In addition, there is marked thickening and abnormal signal of the endometrial complex (E) in this patient with early stage endometrial carcinoma. (b) Sagittal T2-weighted MRI in a different patient shows the presence of an adenomyoma (arrows) in the ventral myometrium. This can be differentiated from a leiomyoma by the absence of mass effect on the endometrium and serosal surface of the uterus, its elliptical shape and poorly defined margins. (c) Transverse T2-weighted MRI in a patient with cystic adenomyosis (arrows). The differentiation between cystic adenomyosis and a leiomyoma with central hemorrhage can be difficult. Features favoring cystic adenomyosis include, ill-defined borders with the myometrium, a thick hypointense rim and an elliptical shape. (Figure 3.10 (b) reprinted with permission from Wiley-Liss, New York. See Ref. 15.)

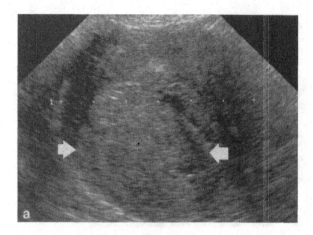

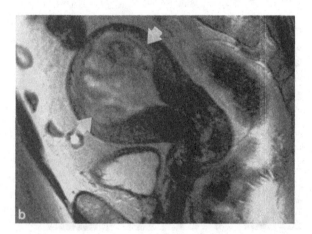

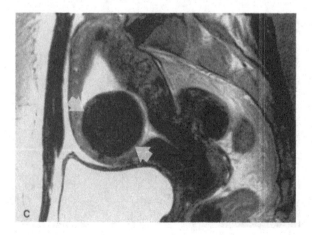

particularly if the uterus is myomatous or the ovaries small as in the postmenopausal patient (Figure 3.12). Differentiating pedunculated leiomyomas from adnexal masses requires the demonstration of continuity with the adjacent myometrium or myometrial vessels, and the absence of a fat plane on T1-weighted sequences between the uterus and the mass. Although it has been suggested that an irregular margin of a uterine leiomyoma at MRI is suggestive of *sarcomatous transformation*, the specificity of this finding has not been established (Figure 3.13).[1] Confident diagnosis of leiomyosarcoma is not possible, unless there is clear evidence of local spread. The most reliable sign for sarcomatous transformation is a rapidly growing myometrial-based mass, particularly in the postmenopausal patient.

Imaging pre-and post-uterine artery embolization

The indications and technique for uterine artery embolization are discussed elsewhere in this text. This chapter will focus on the role of imaging before and after uterine artery embolization (UAE). The type of imaging performed before UAE will vary by center, and will be largely dictated by the locally accepted inclusion and exclusion criteria. Most studies have based their results primarily on US findings, which can be limited by substantial interobserver

Figure 3.11. Endometrial polyp vs. submucosal leiomyoma. (a) Transverse oblique hysterosonography demonstrates a large echogenic mass (arrows) arising from the uterus. The origin, i.e., myometrial versus endometrial is unclear. (b) Sagittal T2-weighted magnetic resonance imaging (MRI) in the same patient confirms the mass (arrows) to be endometrial based. Histology confirmed the mass to be a benign endometrial polyp. (c) Sagittal T2-weighted MRI in a different patient shows a submucosal leiomyoma (arrows) arising from the ventral myometrium for comparison. (Figures 3.11(b) reprinted with permission from Wiley-Liss, New York. See Ref. 15, and Figure 3.11(c) reprinted with permission from Reinhold C, Tafazoli F (1999). See Ref. 8.)

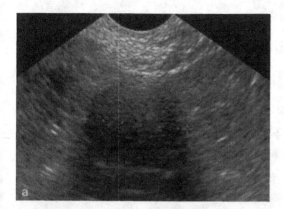

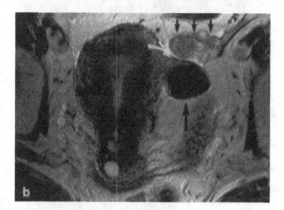

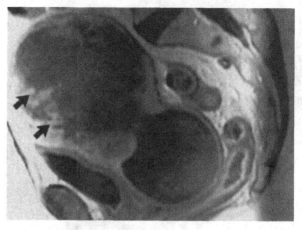

Figure 3.13. Sarcoma. Sagittal T1-weighted magnetic resonance imaging post contrast administration shows a large bilobed mass within the uterus. Note the irregular border (arrows) between the mass and ventral myometrium consistent with a malignant process. (Reprinted with permission from Wiley-Liss, New York. See Ref. 15.)

Figure 3.12. Adnexal mass vs. subserosal leiomyoma. (a) Transverse endovaginal ultrasound shows a hypoechoic mass (calipers) immediately contiguous to the uterus in the left adnexa. A left ovary could not be identified. The differential diagnosis includes a subserosal leiomyoma or ovarian fibrothecoma. (b) Transverse T2-weighted magnetic resonance imaging shows splaying of the myometrium (curved arrow) around the subserosal leiomyoma (large arrow). Note the presence of a normal left ovary (small arrows) separate from the mass.

variability, particularly when estimating the size of large leiomyomas. Leiomyoma size, position, and uterine volume are more accurately delineated with use of MRI. MRI is also superior at diagnosing comorbid disease such as adenomyosis, which can be missed by US,[21,24] or in diagnosing a malignant uterine mass. Imaoka et al.[25] found MRI to have a

sensitivity of 83%, a specificity of 92%, and an accuracy of 89% in distinguishing malignant from benign central uterine masses. In addition to patient selection, a pre-embolization MRI may give some indication concerning the presumed susceptibility to embolization. For example, smaller baseline leiomyoma size and submucosal location are more likely to result in a positive imaging outcome.[26] Leiomyomas with central necrosis associated with hyaline degeneration may respond less successfully to embolization therapy, whereas increased cellularity may result in a better response.

In addition to the pre-treatment evaluation, MRI is ideal for monitoring leiomyomas after embolization therapy. Monitoring the evolution of embolized leiomyomas with US is not accurate, since standardized views from one examination to the next are difficult to reproduce. Katsumori et al.[27] showed the chronological change in relative vascularity of the myomas and uterus after embolization with gelatin sponge particles. Successful embolization resulted in ischemia and avascularity of the myomas both in the acute and chronic phase, while collateral circulation

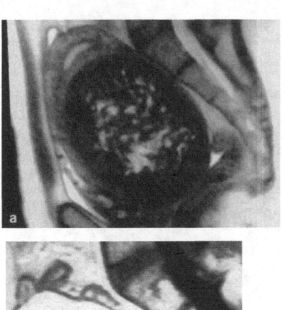

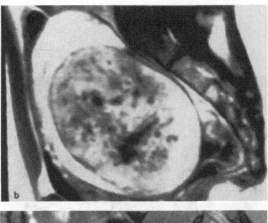

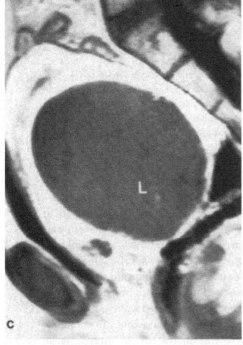

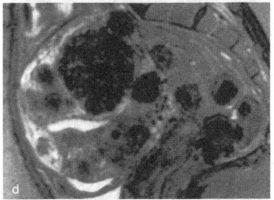

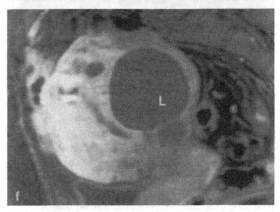

Figure 3.14. Uterine artery embolization (UAE). Sagittal (a,d) T2-weighted and (b,e) T1-weighted contrast enhanced magnetic resonance images in two different patients before UAE. (c,f) Sagittal T1-weighted contrast enhanced magnetic resonance images in the two patients after UAE demonstrate complete avascularity of the leiomyomas (L) indicating successful embolization. A significant decrease in tumor volume can be seen several months after embolization. (Figures 3.14 (a,c) reprinted with permission from Jha et al. (2000). See Ref. 13; Figures 3.14 (d–f) courtesy Dr. S. McCarthy, Yale New Haven Hospital, Connecticut, USA).

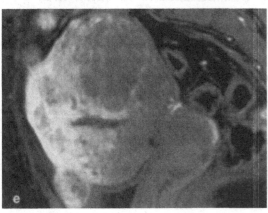

in the normal uterine muscle layer developed within one week (Figure 3.14).[14] A positive correlation has been demonstrated between avascularity of the myomas post embolization and eventual decrease in tumor volume. In addition to avascularity on gadolinium enhanced MRIs, increased signal on non-enhanced T1-weighted sequences due to hemorrhagic necrosis and the presence of blood breakdown products are frequently seen. Necrotic areas containing fluid and air can be present within a leiomyoma after UAE, and should not be mistaken for infection. The mean reduction of myoma volume at two and six months have been reported ranging from 20% to 43% and 52% to 59%, respectively.[28,29,30]

Conclusion

Imaging plays an important role in: (1) the initial evaluation of patients with suspected uterine leiomyomas; (2) patient selection for appropriate therapeutic strategies; and (3) monitoring treatment response. The type of imaging modality to be used will depend on the particular clinical indication, local availability, and expertise.

REFERENCES

1. Murase E, Siegelman ES, Outwater EK, Perez-Jaffe LA & Tureck RW (1999). Uterine leiomyomas: histopathologic features, MR imaging findings, differential diagnosis, and treatment. *Radiographics* 19: 1179–97.

2. Karasick S, Lev-Toaff AS & Toaff ME (1992). Imaging of uterine leiomyomas. *Am J Roentgenol* 158: 799–805.

3. Salem S (1998). The uterus and adnexa. In *Diagnostic Ultrasound*, ed. Rumack CM, Wilson SR & Charboneau JW, 2nd edn, pp. 535–40. St. Louis, MO: Mosby-Year Book.

4. Dudiak CM, Turner DA, Patel SK, Archie JT, Silver B & Norusis M (1988). Uterine leiomyomas in the infertile patient: preoperative localization with MR imaging versus US and hysterosalpingography. *Radiology* 167: 627–30.

5. Pellerito JS, McCarthy SM, Doyle MB, Glickman MG & DeCherney AH (1992). Diagnosis of uterine anomalies: relative accuracy of MR imaging, endovaginal sonography, and hysterosalpingography. *Radiology* 183: 795–800.

6. Reinhold C, Tafazoli F & Wang L (1998). Imaging features of adenomyosis. *Hum Reprod Update* 4: 337–49.

7. Reinhold C, McCarthy S, Bret PM, Mehio A, Atri M, Zakarian R, Glaude Y, Liang L & Seymour RJ (1996). Diffuse adenomyosis: comparison of endovaginal US and MR imaging with histopathologic correlation. *Radiology* 199: 151–8.

8. Reinhold C, Tafazoli F, Mehio A, Wang L, Atri M, Siegelman ES & Rohoman L (1999). Uterine adenomyosis: endovaginal US and MR imaging features with histopathologic correlation. *Radiographics* 19: S147–60.

9. Schwartz LB, Panageas E, Lange R, Rizzo J, Comite F & McCarthy S (1994). Female pelvis: impact of MR imaging on treatment decisions and net cost analysis. *Radiology* 192: 55–60.

10. Weinreb JC, Barkoff ND, Megibow A & Demopoulos R (1990). The value of MR imaging in distinguishing leiomyomas from other solid pelvic masses when sonography is indeterminate. *Am J Roentgenol* 154: 295–9.

11. Togashi K, Nishimura K, Itoh K et al. (1988). Adenomyosis: diagnosis with MR imaging. *Radiology* 166: 111–14.

12. Walsh JW, Taylor KJ & Rosenfield AT (1979). Gray scale ultrasonography in the diagnosis of endometriosis and adenomyosis. *Am J Roentgenol* 132: 87–90.

13. Jha RC, Ascher SM, Imaoka I & Spies JB (2000). Symptomatic fibroleiomyomata: MR imaging of the uterus before and after uterine arterial embolization. *Radiology* 217: 228–35.

14. Katsumori T, Nakajima K & Hanada Y (1999). MR imaging of a uterine myoma after embolization. *Am J Roentgenol* 172: 248–9.

15. Reinhold C, Gallix BP & Ascher SM (1997). Uterus and cervix. In *MRI of the Abdomen and Pelvis*, ed. Semelka RC, Ascher SM & Reinhold C, pp. 585–660. New York: Wiley-Liss.

16. Siegelman ES & Outwater EK (1999). Tissue characterization in the female pelvis by means of MR imaging. *Radiology* 212: 5–18.

17. Schwartz LB, Zawin M, Carcangiu ML, Lange R & McCarthy S (1998). Does pelvic magnetic resonance imaging differentiate among the histologic subtypes of uterine leiomyomata. *Fertil Steril* 70: 580–7.

18. Novak ER & Woodruff TD (1979). *Novak's Gynecologic and Obstetric Pathology With Clinical and Endocrine Relations*, 8th edn, pp. 260–79. Philadelphia: Saunders.

19. Okizuka H, Sugimura K, Takemori M, Obayashi C, Kitao M & Ishida T (1993). MR detection of degenerating uterine leiomyomas. *J Comp Ass Tomogr* 17: 760–6.

20. Kawakami S, Togashi K, Konishi I, Kimura I, Fukuoka M, Mori T & Konishi J (1994). Red degeneration of uterine

leiomyoma: MR appearance. *J Comp Ass Tomogr* **18**: 925–8.

21. Togashi K, Ozasa H, Konishi I, Itoh H, Nishimura K, Fujisawa I, Noma S, Sagoh T, Minami S, Yamashita K, Nakano Y, Konishi J & Mori T (1989). Enlarged Uterus: differentiation between adenomyosis and leiomyoma with MR imaging. *Radiology* **171**: 531–4.

22. Hricak H, Finck S, Honda G & Göranson H (1992). MR imaging in the evaluation of benign uterine masses: value of gadopentetate dimeglumine-enhanced T1-weighted images. *Am J Roentgenol* **158**: 1043–50.

23. Reinhold C & Khalili I (2002). Postmenopausal bleeding: value of imaging. *Radiol Clin N Am* **40**: 527–62.

24. Arnold LL, Ascher SM, Schruefer JJ, et al. (1995). The nonsurgical diagnosis of adenomyosis. *Obstet Gynecol* **86**: 461–5.

25. Imaoka I, Sugimura K, Masui T, et al. (1999). Abnormal uterine cavity: differential diagnosis with MR Imaging. *Magn Reson Imaging* **17**: 1445–55.

26. Spies JB, Roth AR, Jha RC, Gomez-Jorge J, Levy EB, Chang TC & Ascher SA (2002). Leiomyomata treated with uterine artery embolization: factors associated with successful symptom and imaging outcome. *Radiology* **222**: 45–52.

27. Katsumori T, Nakajima K & Tokuhiro M (2001). Gadolinium-enhanced MR imaging in the evaluation of uterine fibroids treated with uterine artery embolization. *Am J Roentgenol* **177**: 303–7.

28. Pelage JP, Le Dref O, Soyer P, Kardache M, Dahan H, Abitbol M, Merland JJ, Ravina JH & Rymer R (2000). Fibroid-related menorrhagia: treatment with superselective embolization of the uterine arteries and midterm follow-up. *Radiology* **215**: 428–31.

29. Burn PR, McCall JM, Chinn RJ, Vashisht A, Smith JR & Healy JC (2000). Uterine fibroleiomyoma: MR imaging appearances before and after embolization of uterine arteries. *Radiology* **214**: 729–34.

30. Goodwin SC, Bonilla SM, Sacks D, Reed RA, Spies JB, Landow WJ & Worthington-Kirsch RL (2001). Reporting standards for uterine artery embolization for the treatment of uterine leiomyomata. *J Vasc Interv Radiol* **12**: 1011–20.

4

Abdominal myomectomy

Joseph S. Sanfilippo, and Michael Haggerty

The University of Pittsburgh, Pennsylvania, USA

Introduction

It is estimated that approximately 25% of women in the reproductive age have uterine leiomyomas. Even more convincing is that autopsy studies show an incidence as high as 75%.[1,2] Uterine leiomyoma is responsible for a hysterectomy in up to 1.7 million women.[3] Women of reproductive age who have symptomatic myomas have a number of alternative approaches of treatment available to them including abdominal myomectomy, laparoscopic myomectomy, laparoscopic assisted myomectomy, which includes a mini-laparotomy for uterine repair, and hysteroscopic resection, plus a host of other approaches such as freezing, i.e., cryomyolysis, as well as utilization of high energy sources for destruction of the myoma.

Most importantly, clinicians should be aware of current thinking regarding myomas from a number of perspectives including cytogenetics, hormonal effects, growth factor effects, and also extracellular matrix related factors.

With respect to cytogenetics, there is evidence that myomas are three to nine times more frequent in black than in white women. This information suggests a probable genetic pre-disposition.[4] While a specific gene has not been clearly identified, chromosomal analysis of uterine myomas has revealed non-random tumor specific cytogenetic abnormalities in up to 40% of specimens evaluated.[5] Multiple genetic loci have been proposed in the pathogenesis of leiomyomas.

Estrogen and progesterone have an effect on myoma growth following onset of menopause.[1] More specifically, leiomyomas express increased concentrations of aromatase cytochrome P450 mRNA with an associated lower rate of conversion of estradiol to estrone. Independent investigators have noted that both estrogen and progesterone receptors are in increased concentrations over myomas compared to adjacent myometrium.[6,7] The menstrual cycle day(s) also appears to play a role with respect to mitotic activity in that there is increased activity during the secretory phase of the cycle when progesterone levels are elevated.[8] Other researchers have noted that myomas have an increased expression of specific proteins, i.e., BCL-2 which is involved in apoptosis – programmed cell death.[9]

Other elements effecting myomas include growth factors. The epidermal growth factor (EGF) that is involved in mitogenesis is expressed via EGFmRNA protein throughout the menstrual cycle. EGF appears to be an important growth factor with respect to development and proliferation of leiomyomas.[10]

Insulin-like growth factors I and II (IGF-I, IGF-II) that are small polypeptides integrated into cellular proliferation and differentiation also are involved with myoma development. IGF-I mRNA is detected in the myometrium. High affinity IGF receptors have also been identified on uterine myomas as well as normal myometrial membranes.[11] Other factors include platelet-derived growth factor and transforming growth factor beta.[12,13] Heparin-binding growth factors, which include platelet derived growth factor, fibroblast growth factor, vascular endothelial growth factor, plus heparin-binding epidermal growth factor are involved in myoma formation.

Extracellular matrix factors are also involved and consist mainly of interstitial collagens, proteoglycans and fibronectin. These factors appear to be related to growth of myomas and may be involved with the mechanism of action of gonadotropin-releasing hormone agonist treatment and suppression of myoma growth.[14]

The origin of myomas is felt to be smooth muscle cells, either from the uterine muscle or the vasculature supplying the uterus. Presence of a myoma affects the vasculature of the endometrium, which can be related to infertility and menstrual abnormalities, i.e., menorrhagia as well as metrorrhagia. As a myoma grows, it can obstruct the uterine vasculature especially when the myoma is located intramurally. This has been associated with the development of endometrial venule ectasia. The engorged vessels then result in thin atrophic endometrium that overlies a submucous myoma, which can contribute to heavy bleeding.

The risk of malignant transformation of benign leiomyomas remains extremely rare. Of interest, 0.29% of myomas have been reported to undergo malignant change. In a review of 13 000 myomas by Montague and co-workers at Johns Hopkins, 38 cases (0.29%) were noted to have malignant change.[15]

Leiomyomatosis peritonealis disseminata is an unusual entity characterized by multiple small nodules composed of benign smooth muscle cells, fibroblasts, and myofibroblasts as well as decidual cells. They can implant both on the peritoneal surface of the abdomen and travel through the lymphatics. In general leiomyomatosis peritonealis disseminata is a benign self-limited process. Histopathologically myomas have a characteristic whorl-like appearance in contrast to leiomyosarcomas that have traditionally been noted to have a "raw pork" appearance secondary to increased mitotic activity, necrosis, friability, and hemorrhage.

Clinical presentation

The vast majority of patients are asymptomatic; however, symptoms associated with myomas relate in large part to the location of the tumor, size as well as associated degenerative changes. Pain is more common with pedunculated myomas especially when the pedicle undergoes torsion. Pain may also be associated with cervical dilation as with a submucous myoma as it emerges through the lower uterine segment.

It is estimated that 20–50% of myomas are symptomatic.[16] The primary symptoms associated with myomas include menorrhagia, infertility, pregnancy wastage plus pelvic pain and pelvic pressure symptoms. Overall the most common presenting symptom is menorrhagia that occurs with approximately 30% of fibroids. The mechanism of menorrhagia with myomas is believed to be due to ulceration over the submucous myoma that results in abnormal bleeding. To determine the myoma type, the clinician may hysteroscopically assess the angle of the myoma with the adjacent endometrium or perform sonohysterography. In addition, there is data to suggest that fibroids may affect contractility of the uterus. This however may be secondary to blood loss.[17]

Fibroids may cause compression of the venous plexus of the adjacent myometrium and endometrium. This obstruction results in development of venous lakes in the endometrium all of which contribute to abnormal uterine bleeding. Prostaglandins as well as endorphins play a role in the etiology of menorrhagia.[18]

Myomas may also be associated with infertility. Between 27% and 40% of women with multiple myomas are reported to be infertile.[19] Degeneration of uterine myomas is not uncommon. It includes hemorrhagic, hyaline, carneous and caseous degeneration. Degeneration is accompanied by pain and it occurs more commonly during pregnancy.

Clinicians must be concerned when there is ureteral obstruction secondary to enlargement of the uterine fibroids. This can result in hydroureter as well as hydronephrosis. Rectal pressure is rare unless the myoma is incarcerated in the cul de sac or is a large posterior wall myoma directly compressing the rectosigmoid area.

Treatment options

Most women with leiomyomas are asymptomatic and can be followed without treatment. Return visits are scheduled every 6–12 months to assess any changes in growth or the development of symptoms. A rapid growth rate may suggest malignancy and require possible intervention; malignant transformation is rare, occurring in fewer than 0.1% of women with myomas.[20]

Treatment is usually reserved for symptomatic leiomyomas. Type of treatment depends on the presenting symptoms, size, and number, location of leiomyomas, patient's age, future reproductive desires, and the skills and training of the surgeon. Therapy can be medical, surgical, or radiologic interventional embolization. Surgical options include hysterectomy, hysteroscopic myomectomy, laparoscopic myomectomy, and abdominal myomectomy. Because there is no inexpensive long-term medical treatment devoid of acute and chronic side effects, most symptomatic leiomyomas are still managed surgically. Hysterectomy continues to be the most common therapy and often is the treatment of choice if childbearing is completed. This generally provides a cure for the patient and eliminates the risk of recurrence. Hysteroscopic myomectomy is an effective procedure for submucosal leiomyomas. Laparoscopic myomectomy is a minimally invasive technique with advantages of decreased length of stay and decreased convalescence. This is a technically demanding procedure and patient selection is crucial. Some authorities recommend this procedure be limited to one or two leiomyomas and size not greater than 8 cm.[21] Uterine artery embolization is a relatively new alternative to surgery. Long-term effects and proper patient selection remain a point of discussion.

Abdominal myomectomy may well be an excellent option for women who desire future childbearing or who wish to retain their uterus. With multiple leiomyomas, deep intramural involvement or a significantly enlarged uterus, abdominal myomectomy is the treatment of choice. The abdominal incision, operative time, blood loss, and hospital stay are similar to those for hysterectomy.[22]

Preoperative evaluation

Uterine leiomyomas are often found on routine physical examination, during radiologic procedures, or during a workup for pelvic pain and/or mass. Goals are to decide if the symptoms are secondary to a leiomyoma, if surgery is required, and if so what procedure. Symptoms such as abnormal uterine bleeding, acute and chronic pelvic pain, abdominal distension or pressure, urinary and gastrointestinal symptoms, and the findings of a pelvic mass must be thoroughly and appropriately evaluated. Additional preoperative evaluation prior to abdominal myomectomy includes ordering the proper imaging studies, assessing hematologic status, addressing possible gonadotropin-releasing hormone agonist therapy and thorough patient counseling.

Transvaginal or abdominal sonography are excellent first line diagnostic modalities in determining the size, location and number of leiomyomas. In most cases, ultrasound is the only imaging test needed (Figures 4.1 and 4.2). When clinical symptoms such as abnormal bleeding are encountered, ultrasonography is also extremely useful in initial evaluation of the endometrial cavity. Emanuel demonstrated that a thin endometrial stripe and the absence of a leiomyoma near the endometrial cavity is strongly associated with a negative hysteroscopic examination.[23] If these requirements are not met further evaluation with sonohysterography or hysteroscopy is indicated (Figures 4.3, 4.4 and 4.5, see also color plates). The diagnosis of a submucous leiomyoma will require the addition of hysteroscopic myomectomy to the scheduled abdominal

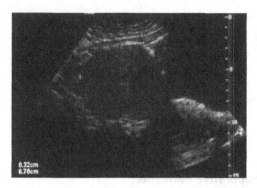

Figure 4.1. Pedunculated leiomyoma. Transabdominal ultrasound: transverse view of the uterus demonstrates a fundal pedunculated leiomyoma measuring 8.3 × 6.8 × 10.6 cm.

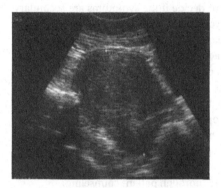

Figure 4.2. Intramural leiomyoma. Transvaginal ultrasound: Sagittal view of the uterus demonstrates an anterior, intramural myoma measuring 4.7 × 4.5 × 6.0 cm.

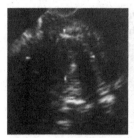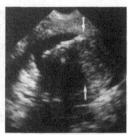

Figure 4.3. Submucosal leiomyoma. (a) Transvaginal ultrasound: sagittal view shows a uterine leiomyoma; (b) sonohysterography: the leiomyoma is found to be intracavitary. Reprinted from Gynecologic Imaging, John C. Anderson, p. 206. (1999), by permission of Churchill Livingstone.

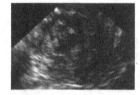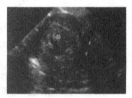

Figure 4.4. Intramural leiomyoma. (a) Transvaginal ultrasound: a leiomyoma (asterisk) is visualized but its relationship to the uterine cavity is unclear; (b) sonohysterography with a fluid filled cavity (arrowheads) demonstrates the leiomyoma to be intramural. Reprinted from Gynecologic Imaging, John C. Anderson, p. 205, (1999), by permission of Churchill Livingstone.

myomectomy. Magnetic resonance imaging (MRI) is very useful in cases where ultrasound is suboptimal secondary to multiple leiomyomas, marked uterine enlargement, or to differentiate a leiomyoma from an adnexal mass (Figure 4.6). MRI may also be helpful in differentiating adenomyosis from leiomyomas, which often exhibit similar clinical and physical findings. Endometrial sampling to evaluate abnormal uterine bleeding should be done when appropriate.

Prior to surgery hematologic status must be evaluated. Approximately 30% of myomectomy patients have menorrhagia. These chronic episodes of heavy vaginal bleeding often lead to iron-deficiency anemia. These patients require oral iron supplements, such as ferrous sulfate 325 mg three times a day. Folate, used in DNA synthesis and therefore in erythropoesis, is often depleted by menorrhagia. Folate can be administered orally in 1 mg per day supplements. These hematinics often require several months to return serum hemoglobin levels to normal.

Sometimes the vaginal bleeding is so severe or prolonged that iron therapy alone will not allow adequate elevation of the patient's hemoglobin. In these scenarios a gonadotropin-releasing hormone agonist to induce amenorrhea is often effective in combination with iron therapy. Gonadotropin-releasing hormone agonists (GnRHa) suppress the hypothalamic–pituitary axis thereby decreasing ovarian function and causing a hypoesterogenic

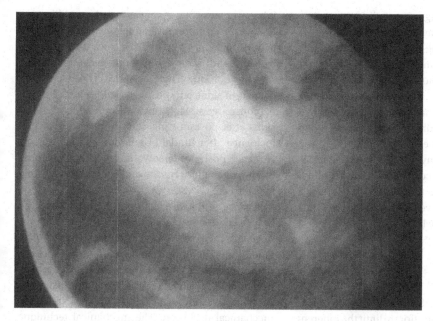

Figure 4.5. Hysteroscopy demonstrates a submucosal leiomyoma. See also color plates.

state. This typically results in a 50% maximum reduction in fibroid and overall uterine volume.[24] This hypoestrogenic state induces endometrial atrophy that relieves the heavy vaginal bleeding. After GnRHa therapy is stopped there is regrowth of the uterus and fibroids to pretreatment size.[25] Stovall in a randomized, double-blinded, placebo-controlled study concluded that GnRHa plus iron therapy is more effective in treating anemia than iron alone. In this study one patient group received leuprolide acetate 3.75 mg monthly for three injections and ferrous sulfate 525 mg orally twice daily. The other group received placebo injections and iron therapy. At the end of three months, 74% of the agonist-iron treated patients had a hemoglobin level greater than or equal to 12 g/dl compared to 46% of the placebo-iron group.[26] Other potential benefits attributed to GnRHa therapy are improvement in pelvic pain, reduced intraoperative blood loss and the ability to convert a planned midline incision into a transverse incision.[27] Because of the hypoestrogenic state produced by GnRHa therapy several side effects can be exhibited. These

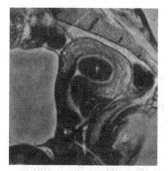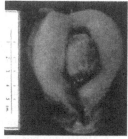

Figure 4.6. Submucosal leiomyoma. (a) Magnetic resonance imaging through the midline of the uterus shows a submucosal leiomyoma (F) surrounded by endometrium; (b) gross specimen. Reprinted from *Gynecologic Imaging*, John C. Anderson, p. 252, (1999), by permission of Churchill Livingstone.

include hot flashes, headaches, and vaginal dryness. Although GnRHa can cause a decrease in bone mineral density, short-term therapy limited to three to six months avoids significant changes. In summary, GnRHa therapy has a role in preoperative therapy but its use must be individualized.

Preoperative counseling must outline the potential complications that may occur during abdominal myomectomy and the long-term reproductive implications. The risks of myomectomy include bleeding requiring blood transfusion, a 2% chance of converting to hysterectomy, infection, and damage to the gastrointestinal or urinary system. Postoperative adnexal or intrauterine adhesions can contribute to infertility and/or spontaneous abortion.

Pregnancy following myomectomy puts the patient at risk for placenta accreta and uterine rupture. If deep myometrial dissection is needed to remove the leiomyoma, an elective cesarean section is currently the best mode of delivery.

Surgical techniques

The surgical techniques for abdominal myomectomy were developed in an effort to limit the inherent risks of blood loss, leiomyoma persistence or recurrence, and formation of adhesions. These techniques can be subdivided into exposure, uterine incision, dissection, and closure of the uterine defect.

Adequate exposure begins with the choice of abdominal incision. Proper exposure enables leiomyoma removal and adequate hemostasis. The majority of abdominal myomectomies can be performed using a Pfannenstiel skin incision and separation of the anterior rectus sheath in a curvilinear cephalad direction. Some experts recommend a Maylard incision when uterine size is greater than 12 weeks.[28] Meticulous hemostasis on entering the peritoneal cavity decreases estimated blood loss and prevents the entrance of blood into the peritoneal cavity that may contribute to adhesion formation. After the peritoneal cavity is entered and any powder has been removed from the operator's gloves, an exploration of the abdominal and pelvic cavity is completed. A self-retaining retractor is then placed if needed and the bowels are packed into the upper abdomen.

The next major decision involves location of the uterine incision, which is determined by the size, number, and distribution of the uterine leiomyomas.

Whenever possible, a single, anterior, midline incision is used to remove all leiomyomas. Adjacent leiomyomas may be mobilized toward the primary incision and removed without making another serosal incision. This incision(s) decreases the chance of adnexal and bowel adhesions. Tulandi demonstrated a 93.7% incidence of adnexal adhesions after posterior incisions compared to a 55% incidence after fundal or anterior wall incisions.[29] However, posterior leiomyomas may require a posterior incision for removal and sometimes multiple incisions are necessary.

Because of the vascularity of the uterus and the time needed to close the uterine defect, several prophylactic measures have been suggested to limit blood loss. The options include dilute vasopressin or mechanical vascular compression. Ginsberg et al. performed a prospective randomized study comparing diluted vasopressin (20 units/20ml of NS) versus mechanical occlusion. The mechanical technique occluded the uterine vessels at the level of the internal os. An avascular area was entered in each broad ligament using a right angle clamp. A penrose drain was passed through the defects and secured with Kelley clamps. The ovarian vessels were occluded bilaterally using atraumatic vascular clamps on both infundibulopelvic ligaments. Their results showed no difference in operative blood loss, operative time, postoperative febrile morbidity, preoperative, and postoperative hematocrits or transfusion rates.[30]

Most myomectomies are performed using dilute vasopressin (20 Units in 40–60cc NS) that is injected into the myometrium surrounding the leiomyoma. The hemostatic effects usually last 30 minutes. Since vasopressin induces vasoconstriction at the vascular bed, intravascular injection is avoided in order to prevent potential systemic effects.

The uterine incision is usually performed with either a knife or bovie. This incision should extend through the serosa, myometrium and into the leiomyoma to be removed (Figure 4.7, see also color plates). The leiomyoma is then grasped with a tenaculum for traction. Allis clamps can be applied to the incised myometrium for additional exposure and hemostasis. A pseudocapsule envelops

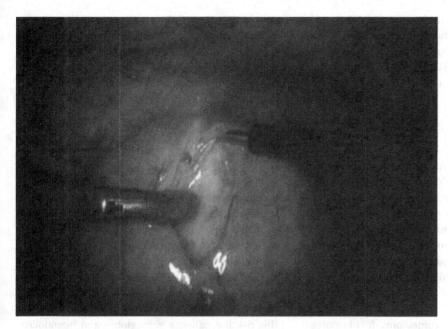

Figure 4.7. Myomectomy. Uterine incision extends through the serosa and myometrium and into the leiomyoma. See also color plates.

the leiomyoma. This false capsule was formed by the leiomyoma compressing the surrounding myometrium. Blunt dissection with a scalpel handle, scissors, or periosteal elevator is used to remove the leiomyoma. By staying between the pseudocapsule and leiomyoma blood loss should be minimal and dissection simplified.

Once the leiomyomas are removed from the initial incision, closure of the uterine defect is accomplished. If the endometrial cavity is entered the myometrium immediately above it is closed with 3–0 or 4–0 synthetic absorbable sutures. The myometrial defect mandates closure of all dead space in order to maintain hemostasis and prevent hematoma formation. Using interrupted figure-of-eight or mattress sutures with 2–0 synthetic, delayed absorbable sutures usually accomplishes this. A multilayer closure is often needed for best results. Once the myometrial defect is repaired serosal closure is performed using a continuous 3–0 or 4–0 absorbable suture in a "baseball" or subcuticular fashion. This minimum suture exposure may lessen the chance of adhesions.

Adhesion prevention

Principles of careful, meticulous hemostasis, least reactive absorbable sutures, copious amounts of irrigation and use of adhesion barriers merit consideration by the gynecologic surgeon.

Adhesion prevention is also related to the location of the incision. Every effort should be made to maximize the efficacy of an incision, i.e., remove as many myomas as possible. As stated above, ideally the incision is located on the anterior surface of the uterus to minimize scarring associated with the fallopian tubes and ovaries. It may be required to dissect the bladder off the uterus as part of the anterior approach. Sawada et al. has reported post-operative adhesion prevention with oxidized-regenerated cellulose adhesion barriers.[31] Patients undergoing myomectomy had the oxidized regenerated cellulose barrier applied. When second look procedures were performed the patients with the barrier had significantly less adhesion formation in comparison to controls. Other barriers have also been utilized including Surgicel and hyaluronic acid. While there is no substitute for meticulous hemostasis and gentle tissue handling, use of barriers should be considered to supplement this approach thus minimizing the chances of adhesion formation.

Surgical outcomes

Abdominal myomectomy was not a common procedure prior to the middle of the twentieth century. Advances in surgical technique have made abdominal myomectomy a safe procedure in women with symptomatic leiomyomas. With more women requesting alternatives to hysterectomy it is important to communicate surgical outcomes during the informed consent discussion. Abdominal myomectomy has demonstrated an 81% success rate in treating menorrhagia.[32] Pelvic pain and dysmenorrhea may be alleviated by myomectomy. It is important for the patient to realize that leiomyomas may coexist with other conditions such as endometriosis, adenomyomas, or pelvic adhesions that may be a source of persistent pain.

The contribution of leiomyomas to infertility and reproductive failure is difficult to assess. To date randomized controlled trials have not been conducted. It appears that leiomyomas, which distort the uterine cavity, may cause infertility and lead to recurrent miscarriages. Removal of these leiomyomas seems to be of benefit but randomized controlled treatment trials are urgently needed.

With uterine conservation the patient must realize there is a risk of leiomyoma recurrence. A series incorporating 622 women who underwent abdominal myomectomy reported a 10 year recurrence rate of 27% using pelvic examination and sonography.[33] Transvaginal ultrasound has demonstrated a recurrence rate of 51%.[34] Fortunately most of these recurrences are asymptomatic. The risk of recurrence is most closely associated with the number of leiomyomas present during the initial surgery. The goal during surgery is to remove all leiomyomas to lower the risk of recurrence. The literature has conflicting data in regard to GnRHa therapy and leiomyoma recurrence.[35,36] The clinically relevant information includes the potential risk of future surgery after abdominal myomectomy. The need for an additional myomectomy or hysterectomy is 15–18% over the next 10 post-operative years.[37,38]

Complications

As with any surgical procedure, there are risks of complications when performing abdominal myomectomy. Intraoperative findings may require that a hysterectomy be performed. This occurs in approximately 2% of cases and is usually secondary to uncontrollable hemorrhage or inability to reconstruct the uterus after removing multiple leiomyomas. Significant intraoperative blood loss may require the patient to undergo a blood transfusion. To decrease this risk the patient's hemoglobin and hematocrit should be maximized prior to surgery. Intraoperative pitressin use and good surgical techniques also decrease estimated blood loss. Injuries to the adjacent gastrointestinal and urologic systems are potential risks. Postoperative fever is not uncommon and is often the result of extensive tissue trauma. A detailed history and physical examination and appropriate diagnostic tests should rule out an infectious cause such as urinary tract infection, wound infection, pneumonia, and septic pelvic thrombophlebitis. Other sources of fever are atelectasis and deep vein thrombosis. Prophylactic antibiotics are routinely administered preoperatively. Pelvic pain and fever postoperatively may also be associated with a uterine hematoma. A pelvic ultrasound is useful in making the diagnosis. Proper closure of the uterine defect may avoid this complication. Treatment is supportive with analgesics and antibiotics. Pelvic and abdominal adhesions can also be associated with abdominal myomectomy. These adhesions can lead to infertility, pelvic pain, and bowel obstruction. The informed consent process should notify the patient of all the above risks.

REFERENCES

1. Nowak R (1990). Fibroids: Pathophysiology and Current Medical Treatment. Bailliere's *Clin Obst Gynaecol* **13**(2): 223–38.

2. Cramer S & Patel A (1990). The frequency of uterine leiomyomas. *Am J Clin Pathol* **94**: 435–8.

3. Wilcox L, Koonin M, Pokres R, et al. (1994). Hysterectomy in the United States, 1988–1990. *Obstet Gynecol* **83**: 549–55.

4. Cramer D (1992). Epidemiology of myomas. *Semin Reprod Endocrinol* **10**: 320–4.

5. Rein M, Friedman A, Barbari R, et al. (1991). Cytogenetic abnormalities in uterine leiomyomas. *Obstet Gynecol* **77**: 923–6.

6. Ville B, Caharnock-Jones D, Sharke M, et al. (1997). Distribution of A & B forms of the progesterone receptor messenger ribonucleic acid and protein in uterine leiomyoma and adjacent myometrium. *Hum Reprod* **12**: 815.

7. Branden D, Ericson T, Keenan E, et al. (1995). Estrogen receptor gene expression in human uterine leiomyoma. *J Clin Endocrinol Metab* **80**: 1876–81.

8. Kawaguchi D, Fujii S & Konishi I (1989). Mitotic activity in uterine leiomyomas during menstrual cycle. *Am J Obstet Gynecol* **160**: 637–41.

9. Matsuo H, Maruo T & Samoto T (1997). Increased expression of BCL-2 protein in human uterine leiomyoma and its regulation by progesterone. *J Clin Endocrinol Metab* **82**: 293–9.

10. Hoffman G, Rao CV, Barrows G, et al. (1984). Binding sites for epidermal growth factor in human uterine tissues and leiomyomas. *J Clin Endocrinol Metab* **58**: 880–4.

11. Ghahary A & Murphy L (1989). Uterine insulin – like growth factor 1 receptor: regulation by estrogen and variations throughout the estrous cycle. *Endocrinology* **125**: 597–604.

12. Fayed Y, Tsibras J, Langenberg P, et al. (1989). Human uterine leiomyoma cells: binding and growth responses to endothelial growth factor, platelet-derived growth factor, and insulin. *Lab Invest* **60**: 30–7.

13. Klagsburn M & Dluz S (1993). Smooth muscle cell and endophilic growth factors. *Trends in Cardiovasc Med* **3**: 213–17.

14. Stewart D, Fredman A, Peck R & Nowak R (1994). Relative overexpression of collagen type I and collagen type II. Messenger RNAs by uterine leiomyoma during the follicular phase of the menstrual cycle. *J Clin Endocrinol Metab* **79**: 900–6.

15. Montague H, Schwartz A & Woodruff J (1965). Carcinoma arising in a leiomyoma of the uterus. *Am J Obstet Gynecol* **92**: 421.

16. Hunt J & Wallach E (1974). Uterine factors in infertility – an overview. *Clin Obstet Gynecol* **17**: 44–64.

17. Lumsden M & Wallace E (1998). Clinical presentation of uterine fibroids. *Bailliere's Clin Obstet Gynaecol* **12**: 177–95.

18. Fraser I, McKaron G, Markham R, et al. (1986). Measured menstrual loss in women with menorrhagia associated with pelvic disease or coagulation disorder. *Obstet Gynecol* **68**: 630–3.

19. Buttram V & Reiter R (1981). Uterine leiomyoma – etiology, symptomatology and management. *Fert Steril* **36**: 433–45.

20. Buttram VC Jr (1986). Uterine leiomyomata-etiology, symptomatology and management. In *Gonadotropin Down-Regulation in Gynecologic Practice*, pp. 275–96. New York: Alan R Liss.

21. Dubuisson JB, Chapron C, Fauconnier A & Kreiker G (1997). Laparoscopic myomectomy and myolysis. *Curr Opin Obstet Gynecol* **9**: 233–8.

22. Iverson RE Jr, Chelmow D, Strohbehn K, Waldman L & Evantash EG (1996). Relative morbidity of abdominal hysterectomy and myomectomy for management of uterine leiomyomas. *Obstet Gynecol* **88**: 415–19.

23. Emanuel MH, Verdel MJ, Wamsteker K, et al. (1995). A prospective comparison of transvaginal ultrasonography and diagnostic hysteroscopy in the evaluation of patients with abnormal uterine bleeding: clinical implications. *Am J Obstet Gynecol* **72**: 547–52.

24. Freidman AJ, Barbieri RL, Benacerraf BR & Schiff I (1987). Treatment of leiomyomata with intranasal or subcutaneous leuprolide, a gonadotropin-releasing hormone agonist. *Fertil Steril* **48**: 560–64.

25. Matta WH, Shaw RW & Nye M (1989). Long-term follow-up of patients with uterine fibroids after treatment with the LHRH agonist buserelin. *Br J Obstet Gynecol* **96**: 200–6.

26. Stovall TG, Muneyyirci-Delale O, Summit RL Jr & Scialli AR (1995). GnRH agonist and iron versus placebo and iron in the anemic patient before surgery for leiomyomas: a randomized controlled trial. *Obstet Gynecol* **86**: 64–71.

27. Lethaby A, Vollenhoven B & Sowter M (1999). Pre-operative gonadotropin-releasing hormone analogue before hysterectomy or myomectomy for uterine fibroids (Cochrane Review). In *The Cochrane Library*, Issue 2. Oxford: Update Software.

28. Thompson JD & Rock JA (1997). Leiomyomata uteri and myomectomy. In *Te Linde's Operative Gynecology*, 8th edn, pp. 731–70. Philadelphia: Lippincott Raven Publishers.

29. Tulandi T, Murray C & Guralink M (1993). Adhesion formation and reproductive outcome after myomectomy and second-look laparoscopy. *Obstet Gynecol* **82**: 213–15.

30. Ginsburg ES, Benson CB, Garfield JM, Gleason RE & Freidman AJ (1993). The effect of operative technique and uterine size on blood loss during myomectomy: a prospective randomized study. *Fertil Steril* **60**: 956–62.

31. Sawada T, Nishizawa H, Nishio E & Kadowaki M (2000). Postoperative adhesion prevention with an oxidized regenerated cellulose adhesion barrier in fertile women. *J Reprod Med* **45**: 387–9.

32. Buttram VC & Reiter RC (1981). Uterine leiomyomata: etiology, symptomatology and management. *Fertil Steril* **36**: 433–45.

33. Candiani GB, Fedele L, Parazzini F & Villa L (1991). Risk of recurrence after myomectomy. *Br J Obstet Gynaecol* **98**: 385–9.

34. Fedele L, Parazzini F, Luchini L, Mezzopane R, Tozzi L & Villa L (1995). Recurrence of fibroids after myomectomy: a transvaginal ultrasonographic study. *Hum Repro* **10**: 1795–6.

35. Fedele L, Vercellini P, Bianchi S, Brioschi D & Dorta M (1990). Treatment of GnRH agonists before myomectomy and the risk of short-term myoma recurrence. *Br J Obstet Gynecol* **97**: 393–6.

36. Friedman AJ, Daly M, Juneau-Norcross M, et al. (1992). Recurrence of myomas after myomectomy in women pretreated with leuprolide acetate depot or placebo. *Fertil Steril* **58**: 205–8.

37. Buttram VC & Reiter RC (1981). Uterine leiomyomata: etiology, symptomatology and management. *Fertil Steril* **36**: 433–45.

38. Acien P & Quereda F (1996). Abdominal myomectomy: results of a simple operative technique. *Fertil Steril* **65**: 41–51.

5

Laparoscopic management of uterine myoma

Daniel S. Seidman,[1] Ceana H. Nezhat,[2] Farr Nezhat,[2] and Camran Nezhat[2]

[1]Chaim Sheba Medical Center, Tel Hashomer Israel
[2]Stanford University School of Medicine, California, USA

The introduction of the laparoscopic approach for the management of intramural and subserosal uterine myomas has to a great extent revolutionized the modern management of myomas. Previously the only way to remove intramural and subserous myomas was by laparotomy, a procedure associated with significant postoperative morbidity.[1] Therefore, physicians traditionally reserved abdominal myomectomy for a selected group of women where the risks and discomfort involved with laparotomy were judged worthy of the potential to preserve and enhance their fertility.[1,2] Studies published in 1999 confirmed the advantages of laparoscopic myomectomy, such as the low morbidity and rapid recovery, which has led to the growing application of the technique towards women with symptomatic uterine myoma.[3,4] However, laparoscopic operation is also associated with potential disadvantages including prolonged anesthesia, increased blood loss and possibly postoperative adhesion formation.[5,6] This has led to a renewed interest in regard to the precise indications for performing laparoscopic myomectomy.[7–14]

Indications

The primary reason for performing myomectomy in women of reproductive age is the preservation of the uterus for the purpose of childbearing. However, an increasing number of women currently elect to undergo laparoscopic removal of myomas, due to various symptoms associated with a rapidly growing or bulky uterus. In addition, some women resort to laparoscopic myomectomy when fibroids that are associated with heavy menstrual bleeding cannot be removed hysteroscopically.

It remains undetermined at present, which women will benefit most from the surgical removal of uterine myomas. Since myomas are common in women who are 35 years of age, a naturally subfertile group, the impact of uterine myomas on fertility remains controversial. However, it has been shown that infertile women with fibroids undergoing assisted reproductive treatment (ART) have a lower pregnancy rate in comparison with matched-age women with no fibroid.[7] Significantly lower implantation and pregnancy rates were found in patients with intramural or submucosal fibroids even when there was no uterine cavity deformation.[7] Furthermore, the pregnancy rate observed within a year of myomectomy is higher than that observed in couples with unexplained infertility with no treatment.[6,8,9]

Pritts[10] recently performed a systematic literature review to determine whether leiomyomata are associated with decreased fertility rates. In her review she identified three prospective studies and eight retrospective studies. All included a control group but none was randomized. Most of the studies dealt with women with unexplained infertility (except for the fibroids) and the success rate of ART (essentially in vitro fertilization (IVF), as determined by the rates of pregnancy, implantation and delivery in relation to the location of the fibroids.[10] Pritts[10] found that when evaluating the outcomes of women with any combination of subserosal, intramural and/or submucosal fibroids, the relative risks (RR) of pregnancy, implantation and delivery rates were 1.02 (95% confidence interval (CI) 0.89–1.17); 0.75 (95% CI 0.63–0.89) and 0.83 (95% 0.68–1.01), respectively, when compared with infertile controls. Only the implantation rates were significantly different. These data included those women undergoing IVF (and in a single study, spontaneous conceptions).

Women with fibroids having no intra-cavitary component (subserosal, intramural, or both) had a RR of pregnancy of 0.96 (95% CI 0.82–1.12), of implantation of 0.86 (95% CI 0.73–1.02) and of delivery of 0.98 (95% CI 0.80–1.19) compared to infertile controls without fibroids.[10] Furthermore, women with only intramural fibroids had RRs of pregnancy, implantation, and delivery of 0.94 (95% CI 0.73–1.20), 0.81 (95% CI 0.60–1.09) and 1.01 (95% CI 0.73–1.34), respectively, when compared with their infertile counterparts without fibroids.

When analyzing the data for women who had submucosal fibroids and abnormal endometrial cavities, significantly lower rates of pregnancy were found compared with their infertile counterparts without fibroids, RR 0.32 (95% CI 0.13–0.70) and implantation, RR 0.28 (95% CI 0.10–0.72).

The analysis for women undergoing resection of submucosal myomas and their subsequent fertility outcomes included those who underwent spontaneous attempts at conception and those utilizing assisted reproduction. There was a significant increase in pregnancy rates in women after myomectomy versus a control group with infertility, but without fibroids, RR 1.72 (95% CI 1.13–2.58). In the study in which delivery rates after resection of submucosal fibroids were evaluated, the relative risks were equivalent to the control group, RR 0.98 (95% CI 0.45–2.41).[10]

Subgroup analysis failed to indicate any effect on fertility of fibroids that did not have a submucous component. Conversely, women with submucous myomas demonstrated lower pregnancy rates (RR 0.30; 95% CI 0.13–0.70) and implantation rates (RR 0.28; 95% CI 0.10–0.72) than infertile controls. Results of surgical intervention were similar. When all fibroid locations were considered together, myomectomy

Table 5.1. Advantages of laparoscopic myomectomy

- Same results as myomectomy by laparotomy in terms of restoring fertility and pregnancy outcome
- Low morbidity
- Rapid recovery
- Short hospital stay
- Improved patient convenience and recovery
- Better assessment of other pelvic pathologies

results were again widely disparate. However, when women with submucous myomas were considered separately, pregnancy was increased after myomectomy compared with infertile controls (RR 1.72; 95% CI 1.13–2.58) and delivery rates were now equivalent to infertile women without fibroids (RR 0.98; 95% CI 0.45–2.41).[10]

Based on the meta-analysis,[10] it was suggested that only myomas with a submucosal or an intracavitary component are associated with decreased reproductive outcomes. However, two prospective matched control studies demonstrated that small intramural fibroids can have a significant negative effect on IVF outcome.[11,12] This is in contrast to previous studies.[13,14] Others have also shown that pregnancy and implantation rates were significantly lower in patients with intramural fibroids even when there was no deformation of the uterine cavity.[7] Pregnancy and implantation rates were not influenced by the presence of subserosal fibroids.[7]

In view of these conflicting studies, multicentre studies must be conducted in order to allow us to determine the precise indications for myomectomy, that is which women will benefit most from the laparoscopic myomectomy.

Advantages and disadvantages

Laparoscopic myomectomy was described in the 1980s and has been repeatedly shown to have some advantages including rapid recovery, short hospitalization, and low morbidity[15–18] (Table 5.1).

A growing amount of indirect evidence currently suggests that following laparoscopic myomectomy

Table 5.2. Reproductive outcome of laparoscopic myomectomy

Authors	Number of Patients	Average number of myomas	Average size of myomas (cm)	Pregnancy rate (%)	Cesarean section rate (%)
Hasson et al.[17]	56	1–9	3–16	26.8	18.2
Dubuisson et al.[55]	21	2	6.2	33.3	80.0
Stringer et al.[43]	5	2	3.6	100	100
Seinera et al.[45]	54	1	4.2	27	80
Miller et al.[57]	40	<5	4–10	75	np
Ribeiro et al.[6]	28	>1	4–13	64	57
Darai et al.[15]	143	1.5	5.4	29	27
Nezhat et al.[4]	115	3	5.9	np	76
Dubuisson et al.[56]	91	2	4.5	53	np
Campo & Garcea[34]	28	1–8	3–8	54	45
Seracchioli et al.[19]	66	≥1	≥5	54	65
Rossetti et al.[58]	26	≥1	5.4	64	74
Dessolle et al.[54]	103	1.7	6.2	41	24

np: not provided.

the pregnancy rate in women with unexplained infertility is fairly good and more than half of subjects become pregnant after surgery (Table 5.2). Only one study has randomly compared laparoscopic and abdominal myomectomy in relation to fertility.[19] No significant differences were found between the two groups in regard to pregnancy rate (55.9% after laparotomy, 53.6% after laparoscopy), abortion rate (12.1 versus 20%), preterm delivery (7.4 versus 5%) and the use of Cesarean section (77.8 versus 65%).[19] Pregnancy outcome in this randomized trial confirmed the validity of the laparoscopic approach as reported in previous reports.

Despite the apparent benefits of the laparoscopic approach for removal of uterine myomas, it seems that at present the technique still demands a high degree of training and skill from the laparoscopic surgeons.[20,21] Furthermore, the technical difficulty in performing laparoscopic morcellation and suturing can result in prolonged time of anesthesia, potentially increased blood loss, and possibly postoperative adhesion formation[5,6] (Table 5.3). These factors seem to limit a wider application of laparoscopic technique.[20]

Table 5.3. Potential disadvantages of laparoscopic myomectomy

- Technically demanding procedure
- Requires a high degree of training and skill
- Expertise in laparoscopic suturing
- Time-consuming due to the need to perform morcellation
- Prolonged time of anesthesia
- Possibly a higher risk of postoperative adhesion formation
- Increased costs with the use of disposable instruments
- Concerns regarding strength of the uterine scar

Laparoscopic myomectomy remains a technically demanding procedure. In the easiest cases, pedunculated myomas may be simply transected, and some enucleated myomas will "pop out" through an incision in the uterine wall. However, in many instances, the incision of intramural myomas is technically challenging. Expertise in laparoscopic suturing is also a crucial requirement for laparoscopic myomectomy.[22]

Dubuisson et al.[23] recently examined the factors that lead to conversion to laparotomy. They found that the risk factors are myoma size of 50 mm as determined by ultrasonography (adjusted OR = 10.3;

95% CI = 2.8–37.9), intramural location of the myomas (adjusted OR = 4.3; 95% CI = 1.3–14.5), anterior location of the myomas (adjusted OR = 3.4; 95% CI = 1.3–9.0) and preoperative use of gonadotropin-releasing hormone (GnRH) agonists (adjusted OR = 5.4; 95% CI = 2.0–14.2).[23]

Laparoscopic myomectomy is usually time-consuming[21] due to the difficulty in morcellating and removing the myoma from the abdominal cavity either through the laparoscopic trocar or a posterior colpotomy. Although subserosal myomas < 5 cm can be managed easily by laparoscopy, larger and intramural lesions require prolonged morcellation and laparoscopic suturing of the uterine defect.

The largest reported myomas removed by laparoscopy have been 15 to 16 cm.[17,18] Some surgeons have suggested that the size of the myoma to be removed laparoscopically should be limited to 10 cm (6) or even 6–7 cm.[24,25] It has also been suggested that no more than four myomas, 3 cm or more in size, should be removed laparoscopically.[24,26]

Concern regarding the strength of the uterine scar following laparoscopic myomectomy is illustrated by 10 case reports of uterine dehiscence during pregnancy.[27–32] The strength of the uterine scar depends on meticulous multilayer suturing of the uterine defect. Failure to do so may lead to the accumulation of an intramural hematoma. Also, the use of the CO_2 laser and electrodesiccation may lead to thermal injury to surrounding tissue and results in poor vascularization and tissue necrosis.[6,18]

Laparoscopic-assisted myomectomy (LAM)

A modification of laparoscopic myomectomy is laparoscopic-assisted myomectomy (LAM) developed by Nezhat et al. in 1994.[33] It has been advocated as a technique that may lessen the concerns regarding laparoscopic myomectomy while retaining the benefits of laparoscopic surgery, namely, short hospital stay, lower costs, and rapid recovery.[33] The decision to proceed with LAM is usually decided in the operating room after the completion of the diagnostic laparoscopy and treatment of any associated pathology. The criteria for LAM are myoma larger than 10–12 cm, or numerous and deep myomas requiring extensive morcellation necessitating uterine repair with sutures.[5]

The procedure is performed after injecting the fibroid's base with 3 to 7 ml of diluted vasopressin in order to minimize blood loss.[5] An incision is made over the uterine serosa until the capsule of the leiomyoma is reached. A corkscrew manipulator is inserted into the leiomyoma and used to elevate the uterus toward the midline suprapubic puncture. With the trocar and manipulator attached to the myoma, the midline 5-mm puncture is enlarged to a 4- to 5-cm transverse incision. Following incision of the fascia transversely at 4–5 cm, the rectus muscles are separated at the midline. The peritoneum is entered transversely, and the leiomyoma is located and brought to the incision using the corkscrew manipulator; a uterine manipulator is used to raise the uterus. The corkscrew manipulator is replaced with two Lahey tenacula. The leiomyoma is shelled sequentially and morcellated, gradually exposing new areas. After complete removal of the leiomyoma, the uterine wall defect is seen through the incision. If uterine size allows, the uterus is brought to the skin through the mini-laparotomy incision to complete the repair. When multiple leiomyomas are found, as many as possible are removed through a single uterine incision. When the leiomyomas are in distant locations and identification is impossible, the minilaparotomy incision is closed temporarily with one layer of running suture or several Allis clamps. The laparoscope is reintroduced, and the leiomyomas are identified and brought to the incision. If posterior leiomyomas are difficult to reach through a minilaparotomy incision, they are removed completely laparoscopically. The uterus is then exteriorized through the minilaparotomy incision.[5]

The uterus is reconstructed in layers using 4-0 to 2-0 and 0 polydioxanone suture without suturing the serosa, and the uterus is palpated to ensure that there are no small intramural leiomyomas. The uterus is returned to the peritoneal cavity, and the fascia and skin are closed in layers. The fascia is closed with 1-0 polyglactin suture and the skin in a subcuticular manner. The laparoscope is used to evaluate the uterus and ensure final hemostasis. The pelvis is evaluated to detect and treat endometriosis and adhesions that may have been obscured previously by myomas. Copious irrigation is performed, and blood clots are removed.

Laparoscopic assisted myomectomy offers several obvious and potential long- and short-term benefits. The major advantages of LAM are ease of repair of the uterus and rapid morcellation of the fibroids. In addition, LAM allows more meticulous suturing of the uterus, thus maintaining better uterine wall integrity.

The results of LAM were compared in patients who had either myomectomy by laparotomy or laparoscopic myomectomy.[33] The myoma weight was significantly greater in the LAM group than in the patients undergoing laparoscopic myomectomy. It was found that LAM could safely replace myomectomy by laparotomy, since patient selection criteria were comparable, and the myoma weights of these two groups were shown to be similar.

When the LAM and laparotomy groups were compared the mean estimated blood loss was found not to be different. However, blood loss among the patients undergoing laparoscopic myomectomy was significantly lower and may be attributed to the smaller myomas removed.[33]

The need to decrease the operating time of laparoscopic myomectomy has been underscored by previous studies.[21] LAM, with conventional morcellation and suturing through the minilaparotomy incisions, allows fast removal of multiple and large myomas, and reduces the duration of the operation. Similar mean operating times for laparoscopic myomectomy and LAM techniques were observed despite larger myomas and their intramural positions, adjunctive laparoscopic procedures, and the smaller incisions in the LAM groups.[33]

Hospitalization after myomectomy by laparotomy was significantly longer than LAM or laparoscopic myomectomy.[33] The hospitalization time is similar for LAM and laparoscopic myomectomy. For both procedures, day surgery is used and the patient usually is discharged on the first postoperative day. The postoperative recovery time is also comparable, despite the differences in the size of the different incisions.[5]

The use of gonadotropin-releasing hormone (GnRH) analogs before laparoscopic myomectomy

Some surgeons have advocated the use of preoperative GnRH agonists (GnRHa) to shrink the fibroids and to facilitate the surgery. However, there are conflicting data on the advantages of such therapy before laparoscopic myomectomy.[26,34] We do not routinely use preoperative GnRH analogs. In fact, Dubuisson et al.[23] found that preoperative use of GnRH agonists increased the risk of conversion from laparoscopy to laparotomy by fivefold (adjusted OR = 5.4; 95% CI = 2.0–14.2).

For women who are anemic, preoperative treatment with GnRHa enables restoration of a normal hematocrit,[35] and reduces the need for transfusion.[36,37] However, the benefits of preoperative GnRHa for laparoscopic myomectomy have recently been challenged in a prospective randomized study.[5] Preoperative GnRHa could soften myomas, causing the identification of surgical cleavage plane difficult and hence lengthening the operative time.[5] Moreover, it may be associated with short-term recurrences of small myomas, which shrink in response to treatment and are therefore missed at surgery.[38,39]

Postoperative complications

Adhesions

Adhesion can be numerous and dense around the sutured uterine incisions.[33] This is an important problem especially when the myomectomy is performed to enhance or preserve fertility. However, data concerning post-surgical adhesion and pregnancy outcome are limited,[40] although some preliminary data are encouraging.[3,4,14,41]

Evaluation of the uterus by second-look laparoscopy after removal of pedunculated and superficial subserosal myomas show complete uterine healing. In contrast, intramural and deep subserosal myomas are associated with evidence of granulation tissue and indentation of the uterus proportional to size of the leiomyoma removed, unless sutures are used to approximate the edges. However, the use of sutures is associated with a higher rate of adhesions.[33] In a study of second-look laparoscopy after myomectomy by laparoscopy, 72 myomectomy sites were checked.[18] The overall rate of postoperative adhesion was 35.6% per patient. The rate of adhesions per myomectomy site was 16.7%. Factors influencing post-myomectomy adhesions are posterior location of the myoma and the existence of sutures.[18] Meticulous suturing techniques facilitated by LAM may therefore reduce the rate of postoperative adhesions.[33]

A recent review of barrier agents for preventing adhesions after surgery for subfertility included 15 randomized controlled trials.[42] Five trials randomized patients while the remainder randomized pelvic organs. Laparoscopy was the primary surgical technique in six trials while the remaining trials were laparotomy. Indications for surgery included myomectomy (five trials), ovarian surgery (four trials), pelvic adhesions (six trials), endometriosis (two trials) and mixed (one trial). Thirteen trials assessed Interceed (TC7, Oxidized Regenerated Cellulose, Ethicon, Inc., Johnson & Johnson Medical Inc.) versus no treatment, two assessed Interceed versus Gore-Tex (W.L. Gore & Associates, Flagstaff, AZ), one trial assessed Gore-Tex versus no treatment.[42] No study reported pregnancy or reduction in pain as an outcome. The absorbable adhesion barrier Interceed was found to reduce the incidence of adhesion formation, both new formation and re-formation, at laparoscopy and laparotomy, but there was insufficient data to support its use to improve pregnancy rates.[42] The summation of the data suggests that Gore-Tex is superior to Interceed in preventing adhesion formation, but it is non-absorbable.[42]

Endometrial-serosal fistula

In patients with intramural fibroids and deep uterine wall defects, endometrial-serosal fistula can occur. At second-look laparoscopy, we have observed indentations at the sites from which myomas have been removed. This was directly proportional to the size of the myomas removed and may therefore represent structural defects. Uteroperitoneal fistu-

las have also been noted following laparoscopic myomectomy.[18] In our opinion, LAM may be a safer approach allowing a meticulous multilayer correction of the uterine defects. However, advancement in laparoscopic skill and instrumentation allows the surgeon to perform laparoscopic suturing of the endometrial cavity in three layers, although the safety of this approach remains to be proven.[43]

Another approach, combined laparoscopic and vaginal myomectomy, has also been suggested in order to treat extensive and deeply infiltrating fundal and posterior wall leiomyomata.[31] The posterior colpotomy permits delivery of the myomas, and allows uterine reconstruction by conventional suturing performed transvaginally. This approach also permits multilayered uterine reconstruction of deep myometrial defects. Similarly, Wang et al.[44] have suggested that laparoscopic-assisted vaginal myomectomy may facilitate hemostasis and uterine repair compared to a purely laparoscopic approach. Here, after laparoscopic inspection and location of uterine myomas, posterior and fundal uterine myomas are removed vaginally.

Ultrasound imaging and Doppler velocimetry have been advocated for studying the evolution of the uterine scar following myomectomy.[45] Sonographic evaluation of the uterine scar may allow detection of alterations in muscular echotexture, but its effectiveness in identifying women at risk of uterine rupture or dehiscence has to be proven.[46]

Uterine rupture

The most severe postoperative complication is uterine rupture during pregnancy. It has been reported in 10 cases after laparoscopic myomectomy.[29–32,47–50] Dubuisson et al.[27] recently reported a follow-up study of 100 patients <45 years of age, who had delivered after laparoscopic myomectomy. The surgery consisted of removal of at least one intramural or subserosal myoma of more than 20 mm diameter. Among these 100 women there were three cases of spontaneous uterine rupture.[27] Because only one of these uterine ruptures occurred on the LM scar, the risk of uterine rupture was determined as 1.0% (95% CI 0.0–5.5%). Seventy-two patients had trials of labor and 58 (80.6%) delivered vaginally. There was no uterine rupture during labor.[27]

Uterine rupture following myomectomy is rare. It is estimated that the incidence is approximately 2% of all pregnancy-related uterine ruptures.[51] Most of the large series to date (Table 5.2) did not confirm the hypothesis that laparoscopic myomectomy is associated with an increased risk for uterine dehiscence during pregnancy. This may also be due to the lack of long-term follow-up of patients who had undergone this surgery rather than the rarity of this complication. It must be remembered that inadequate approximation of the uterine wall and poor healing may predispose patients to uterine rupture.[48]

The use of LAM has been proposed as a means for ensuring that the hysterotomy scars are good.[33] However, this approach does not completely prevent uterine rupture. Two cases have been reported in the literature.[27,30] After our most recent series was published[4] we became aware that two of our patients subsequently had uterine rupture in the third trimester of pregnancy.[32]

A long established dogma dictates that if the endometrial cavity is entered during abdominal myomectomy the patient should undergo cesarean delivery for subsequent pregnancy.[33] Similar guidelines should be followed for laparoscopic myomectomies and LAM. Women with large intramural fibroids, who wish to have children, should be informed about the paucity of data regarding the risk of uterine rupture.

Recurrence

Another concern recently raised is the possibility of incomplete resection of the uterine myomas by laparoscopy leading to the recurrence of myomas.[52,53] In our series[53] there were 38 (33.3%) recurrences after an average interval of 27 months. However, of the 38 women with recurrent myoma only 14 (36.8%) required additional surgery. The cumulative risk of recurrence (Kaplan–Meier curve) was 10.6% after one year, 31.7% after three years, and 51.4% after five years.[53]

The risk of recurrence increases when there is more than one myoma.[52] However, Rossetti et al.[39] reported that neither the number of myomas removed nor the depth of penetration or size were correlated with the risk of recurrence. The use of preoperative GnRHa has been shown to increase the risk of recurrence.[38,39] This may be due to the fact that small fibroids are more likely to be missed during the laparoscopic operation.

In the only randomized study published to date the recurrence of myoma during the follow-up period was similar after myomectomy by laparotomy (22.3%) or by laparoscopy (21.4%).[19] When only large myomata were considered the recurrence rates were 6.7% (laparotomy) and 1.8% (laparoscopy), respectively.[19]

Persistence or recurrence of the myoma after myomectomy may reduce the chances of conception and increase the risks of premature labor. In our view, it is essential to obtain the most complete excision possible. However, it is inevitable that small, undetectable myomata will remain within the myometrium whatever approach is used (laparoscopy or laparotomy).[52]

Conclusion

Laparoscopic myomectomy is currently the procedure of choice for removal of intramural and subserous myomas. The procedure is associated with several advantages including shorter hospital stay, less postoperative pain, and faster recovery, while offering the patient the same results as the conventional myomectomy by laparotomy.

The precise indications justifying laparoscopic removal of uterine myomas remain to be more clearly defined. However, in properly selected patients laparoscopic myomectomy and LAM are a safe and efficient alternative to myomectomy by laparotomy and can be performed in most cases even in the presence of very large myomata.

Laparoscopic myomectomy is a technically demanding procedure requiring special skills such as the ability to perform laparoscopic suturing. LAM, by decreasing these technical demands, and thereby the operative time, may offer a better management, as it allows careful suturing of the uterine defect in layers and avoids excessive electrocoagulation. The adoption of LAM may allow more physicians to offer these advantages to their patients. In any event, due to the possible risk of uterine rupture, patients who conceived after myomectomy should be carefully monitored.

REFERENCES

1. Acien P & Quereda F (1996). Abdominal myomectomy: results of a simple operative technique. *Fertil Steril* **65**: 41–51.
2. Verkauf BS (1992). Myomectomy for fertility enhancement and preservation. *Fertil Steril* **58**: 1–15.
3. Bulletti C, De Ziegler D, Polli V & Flamigni C (1999). The role of leiomyomas in infertility. *J Am Assoc Gynecol Laparosc* **6**: 441–5.
4. Nezhat CH, Nezhat F, Roemisch M, Seidman DS, Tazuke SI & Nezhat CR (1999). Pregnancy following laparoscopic myomectomy: preliminary results. *Hum Reprod* **14**: 1219–21.
5. Seidman DS, Nezhat CH, Nezhat F & Nezhat C (2001). The role of laparoscopic-assisted myomectomy (LAM). *J Soc Laparoendosc Surg* **5**: 299–303.
6. Ribeiro SC, Reich H, Rosenberg J, Guglielminetti E & Vidali A (1999). Laparoscopic myomectomy and pregnancy outcome in infertile patients. *Fertil Steril* **71**: 571–4.
7. Eldar-Geva T, Meagher S, Healy DL, MacLachlan V, Breheny S & Wood C (1998). Effect of intramural, subserosal, and submucosal uterine fibroids on the outcome of assisted reproductive technology treatment. *Fertil Steril* **70**: 687–91.
8. Diczfalusy E & Crosignani PG (1996). Infertility revisited: the state of the art today and tomorrow. *Hum Reprod* **11**: 1779–807.
9. Sudic R, Husch K, Steller J & Daume E (1996). Fertility and pregnancy outcome after myomectomy in sterility patients. *Eur J Obstet Gynecol Reprod Biol* **65**: 209–14.
10. Pritts EA (2001). Fibroids and infertility: a systematic review of the evidence. *Obstet Gynecol Surv* **56**: 483–91.
11. Hart R, Khalaf Y, Yeong CT, Seed P, Taylor A & Braude P (2001). A prospective controlled study of the effect of intramural uterine fibroids on the outcome of assisted conception. *Hum Reprod* **16**: 2411–7.
12. Check JH, Choe JK, Lee G & Dietterich C (2002). The effect on IVF outcome of small intramural fibroids not compressing the uterine cavity as determined by a prospective matched control study. *Hum Reprod* **17**: 1244–8.
13. Dietterich C, Check JH, Choe JK, Nazari A & Fox F (2000). The presence of small uterine fibroids not distorting the endometrial cavity does not adversely affect conception outcome following embryo transfer in older recipients. *Clin Exp Obstet Gynecol* **27**: 168–70.
14. Surrey ES, Lietz AK & Schoolcraft WB (2001). Impact of intramural leiomyomata in patients with a normal endometrial cavity on in vitro fertilization-embryo transfer cycle outcome. *Fertil Steril* **75**: 405–10.
15. Darai E, Dechaud H, Benifla JL, Renolleau C, Panel P & Madelenat P (1997). Fertility after laparoscopic myomectomy: preliminary results. *Hum Reprod* **12**: 1931–4.
16. Dubuisson JB, Chapron C, Verspyck E, et al. (1993). Laparoscopic myomectomy: 102 cases. *Contrac Fertil Sexual* **21**: 920–2.
17. Hasson HM, Rotman C, Rana N, et al. (1992). Laparoscopic myomectomy. *Obstet Gynecol* **80**: 884–8.
18. Nezhat C, Nezhat F, Silfen SL, et al. (1991). Laparoscopic myomectomy. *Int J Fertil* **36**: 275–80.
19. Seracchioli R, Rossi S, Govoni F, Rossi E, Venturoli S, Bulletti C & Flamigni C (2000). Fertility and obstetric outcome after laparoscopic myomectomy of large myomata: a randomized comparison with abdominal myomectomy. *Hum Reprod* **15**: 2663–8.
20. Miskry T & Magos A (1999). Laparoscopic myomectomy. *Semin Laparosc Surg* **6**: 73–9.
21. Shushan A, Mohamed H & Magos AL (1999). How long does laparoscopic surgery really take? Lessons learned from 1000 operative laparoscopies. *Hum Reprod* **14**: 39–43.
22. Tulandi T & al-Took S (1999). Endoscopic myomectomy. Laparoscopy and hysteroscopy. *Obstet Gynecol Clin North Am* **26**: 135–48.
23. Dubuisson JB, Fauconnier A, Fourchotte V, Babaki-Fard K, Coste J & Chapron C (2001). Laparoscopic myomectomy: predicting the risk of conversion to an open procedure. *Hum Reprod* **16**: 1726–31.
24. Mais V, Ajossa S, Guerriero S, Mascia M, Solla E & Melis GB (1996). Laparoscopic versus abdominal myomectomy: a prospective, randomized trial to evaluate benefits in early outcome. *Am J Obstet Gynecol* **174**: 654–8.
25. Parker WH & Rodi IA (1994). Patient selection for laparoscopic myomectomy. *Am Assoc Gynecol Laparosc* **2**: 23–6.
26. Dubuisson JB, Lecuru F, Foulot H, Mandelbrot L, Bouquet de la Joliniere J & Aubriot FX (1992). Gonadotrophin-releasing hormone agonist and laparoscopic myomectomy. *Clin Ther* **14**(Suppl A): 51–6.
27. Dubuisson JB, Fauconnier A, Deffarges JV, Norgaard C, Kreiker G & Chapron C (2000). Pregnancy outcome and deliveries following laparoscopic myomectomy. *Hum Reprod* **15**: 869–73.
28. Foucher F, Leveque J, Le Bouar G & Grall J (2000). Uterine rupture during pregnancy following myomectomy via coelioscopy. *Eur J Obstet Gynecol Reprod Biol* **92**: 279–81.

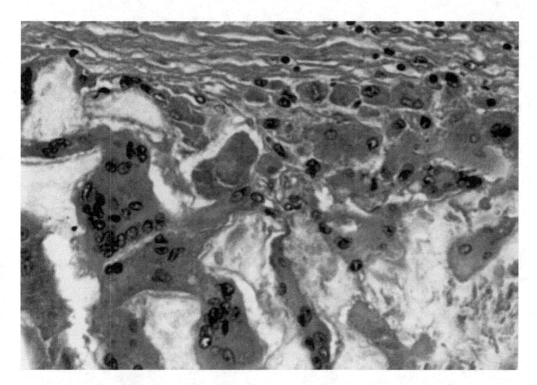

Figure 2.1. Post-embolization specimens characteristically have intravascular foreign body giant cell reaction in peripheral blood vessels. (Hematoxylin and eosin, original magnification × 62.2.)

Figures 2.1 - 17.2 in this section are available for download in colour from www.cambridge.org/9780521184199

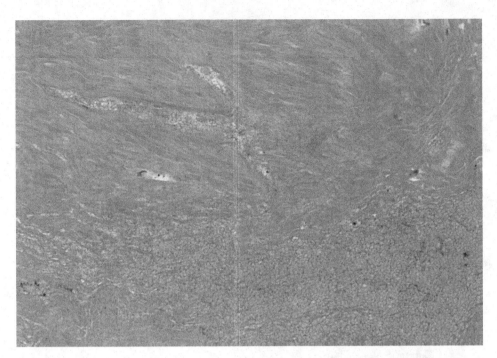

Figure 2.2. This post-embolization myoma has well developed coagulation necrosis characterized by loss of nuclei (karryolysis) and eosinophilia (top of field) and a hemorrhagic zone (bottom). (Hematoxylin and eosin, original magnification × 62.2.)

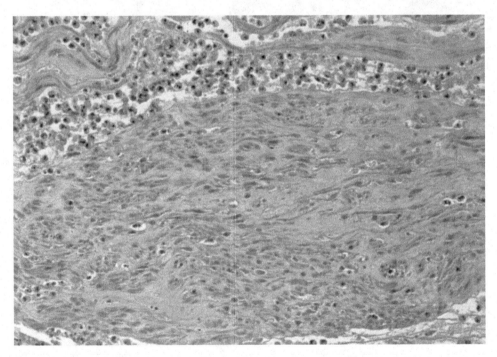

Figure 2.3. Neutrophils infiltrate from the periphery of this infarcted leiomyoma. Necrotic myofibers have well developed coagulation necrosis with cytoplasmic eosinophilia and loss of nuclei (karyolysis). (Hematoxylin and eosin, original magnification × 62.2.)

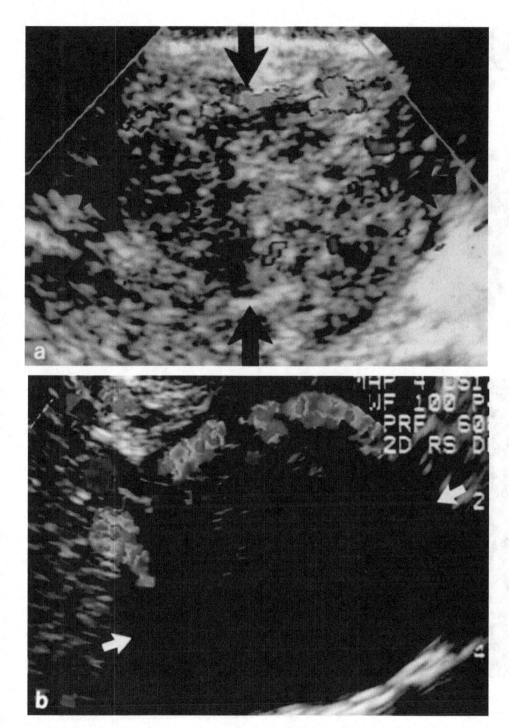

Figure 3.5. Rim of color Doppler. (a) Intramural and (b) subserosal leiomyomas (arrows) in two different patients demonstrate the typical rim of colour Doppler flow with endovaginal ultrasound.

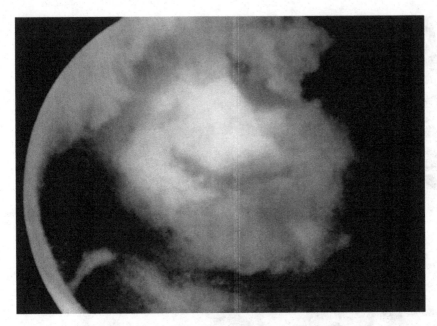

Figure 4.5. Hysteroscopy demonstrates a submucosal leiomyoma.

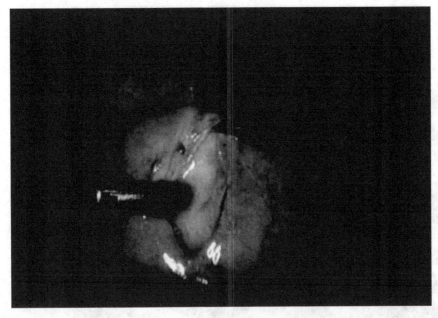

Figure 4.7. Myomectomy. Uterine incision extends through the serosa and myometrium and into the leiomyoma.

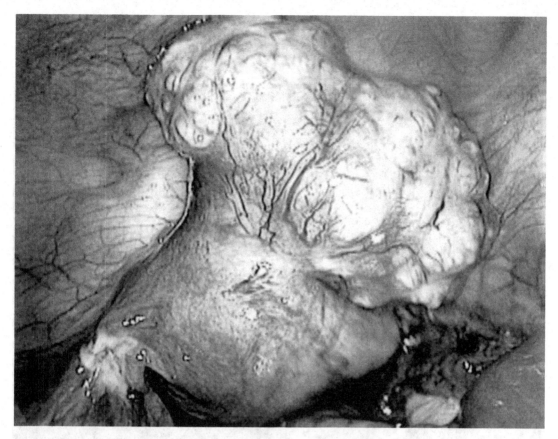

Figure 9.2. Uterus before laparoscopic hysterectomy. A calcified subserous myoma is shown. The patient also had a large cervical myoma (not seen).

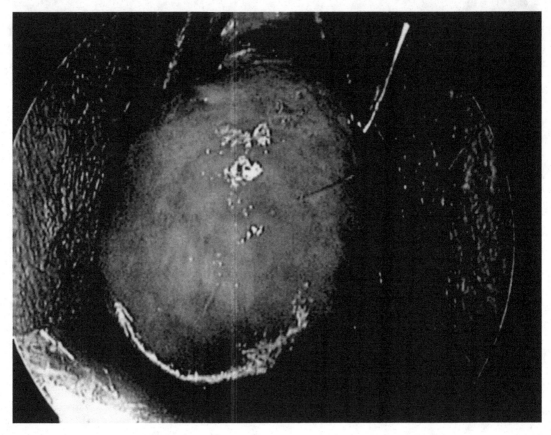

Figure 16.3. A prolapsing submucous myoma.

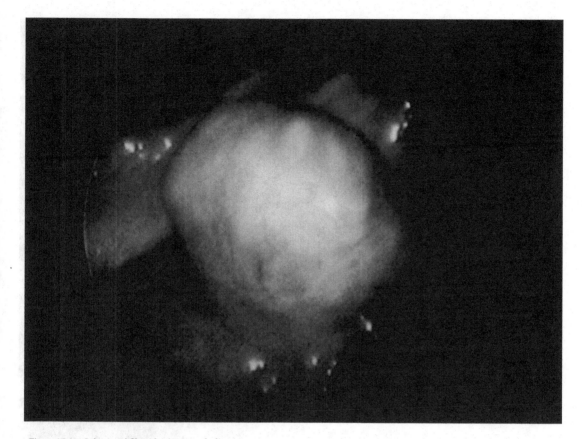

Figure 17.1a. Subserosal fibroid prior to embolization.

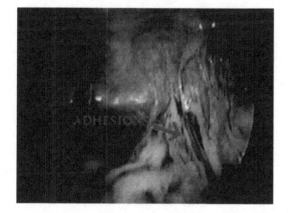

Figure 17.1b. Same patient as for 17.1a two years later.

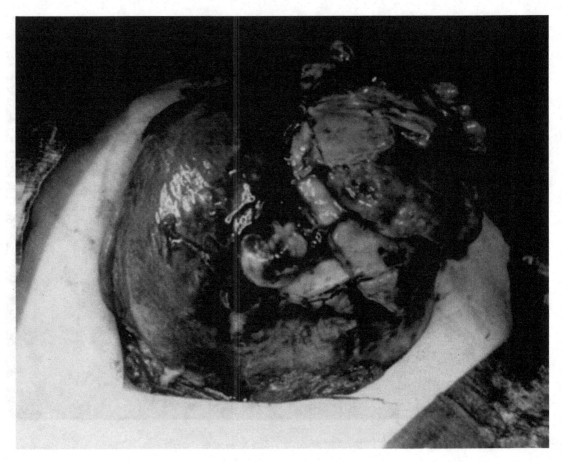

Figure 17.2. Extrusion of infected intramural fibroid following hysterectomy.

29. Friedmann W, Maier RF, Luttkus A, Schafer AP & Dudenhausen JW (1996). Uterine rupture after laparoscopic myomectomy. *Acta Obstet Gynecol Scand* **75**: 683–4.

30. Hockstein S (2000). Spontaneous uterine rupture in the early third trimester after laparoscopically assisted myomectomy. *J Reprod Med* **45**: 139–41.

31. Pelosi MA, 3rd & Pelosi MA (1997). Laparoscopic-assisted transvaginal myomectomy. *J Am Assoc Gynecol Laparosc* **4**: 241–6.

32. Seidman DS, Nezhat CH, Nezhat FR & Nezhat C (2001). Spontaneous uterine rupture in pregnancy 8 years after laparoscopic myomectomy. *J Am Assoc Gynecol Laparosc* **8**: 333–5.

33. Nezhat C, Nezhat F, Bess O, et al. (1994). Laparoscopically assisted myomectomy: A report of a new technique in 57 cases. *Int J Fertil* **39**: 39–44.

34. Campo S & Garcea N (1999). Laparoscopic myomectomy in premenopausal women with and without preoperative treatment using gonadotrophin-releasing hormone analogues. *Hum Reprod* **14**: 44–8.

35. Friedman AJ, Rein NS, Harrison-Atlas D, et al. (1989). A randomized, placebo-controlled, double blind study evaluating leuprolide acetate depot treatment before myomectomy. *Fertil Steril* **52**: 728.

36. Audebert AJM, Madenelat P, Querleu D, et al. (1994). Deferred versus immediate surgery for uterine fibroids: clinical trial results. *Br J Obstet Gynaecol* **101**(Suppl 10): 20–32.

37. Shaw RW (1989). Mechanism of LHRH analogue action in uterine fibroids. *Horm Res* **32**: 150.

38. Fedele L, Pazzarini F, Luchini L, et al. (1995). Recurrence of fibroids after myomectomy: a transvaginal ultrasonographic study. *Hum Reprod* **10**: 1795–6.

39. Rossetti A, Sizzi O, Soranna L, Cucinelli F, Mancuso S & Lanzone A (2001). Long-term results of laparoscopic myomectomy: recurrence rate in comparison with abdominal myomectomy. *Hum Reprod* **16**: 770–4.

40. Seinera P, Arisio R, Decko A, Farina C & Crana F (1999). Laparoscopic myomectomy: indications, surgical technique and complications. *Hum Reprod* **14**: 2460–3.

41. Dubuisson JB, Fauconnier A, Chapron C, Kreiker G & Norgaard C (1998). Second look after laparoscopic myomectomy. *Hum Reprod* **13**: 2102–6.

42. Farquhar C, Vandekerckhove P, Watson A, Vail A & Wiseman D (2000). Barrier agents for preventing adhesions after surgery for subfertility. *Cochrane Database Syst Rev* **2**: CD000475.

43. Stringer NH, Strassner HT, Lawson L, Oldham L, Estes C, Edwards M & Stringer EA (2001). Pregnancy outcomes after laparoscopic myomectomy with ultrasonic energy and laparoscopic suturing of the endometrial cavity. *J Am Assoc Gynecol Laparosc* **8**: 129–36.

44. Wang CJ, Yen CF, Lee CL & Soong YK (2000). Laparoscopic-assisted vaginal myomectomy. *J Am Assoc Gynecol Laparosc* **7**: 510–14.

45. Seinera P, Gaglioti P, Volpi E, Cau MA & Todros T (1999). Ultrasound evaluation of uterine wound healing following laparoscopic myomectomy: preliminary results. *Hum Reprod* **14**: 2460–3.

46. Landi S, Zaccoletti R, Ferrari L & Minelli L (2001). Laparoscopic myomectomy: technique, complications, and ultrasound scan evaluations. *J Am Assoc Gynecol Laparosc* **8**: 231–40.

47. Dubuisson JB, Chavet X, Chapron C, Gregorakis SS & Morice P (1995). Uterine rupture during pregnancy after laparoscopic myomectomy. *Hum Reprod* **10**: 1475–7.

48. Harris WJ (1992). Uterine dehiscence following laparoscopic myomectomy. *Obstet Gynecol* **80**: 545–6.

49. Mecke H, Wallas F, Brocker A & Gertz HP (1995). Pelviscopic myoma enucleation: technique, limits, complications. *Geburtshilfe Frauenheilkd* **55**: 374–9.

50. Pelosi MA, 3rd & Pelosi MA (1997). Spontaneous uterine rupture at thirty-three weeks subsequent to previous superficial laparoscopic myomectomy. *Am J Obstet Gynecol* **177**: 1547–9.

51. Georgakopoulous PA & Bersis G (1981). Sigmoido-uterine rupture in pregnancy after multiple myomectomy. *Int Surg* **66**: 367–8.

52. Fauconnier A, Chapron C, Babaki-Fard K & Dubuisson JB (2000). Recurrence of leiomyomata after myomectomy. *Hum Reprod Update* **6**: 595–602.

53. Nezhat FR, Roemisch M, Nezhat CH, Seidman DS & Nezhat CR (1998). Recurrence rate after laparoscopic myomectomy. *J Am Assoc Gynecol Laparosc* **5**: 237–40.

54. Dessolle L, Soriano D, Poncelet C, Benifla JL, Madelenat P & Darai E (2001). Determinates of pregnancy rate and obstetric outcome after laparoscopic myomectomy for infertility. *Fertil Steril* **76**: 370–4.

55. Dubuisson JB, Chapron C, Chavet X & Gregorakis SS (1996). Fertility after laparoscopic myomectomy of large intramural myomas: preliminary results. *Hum Reprod* **11**: 518–22.

56. Dubuisson JB, Fauconnier A, Chapron C, Kreiker G & Norgaard C (2000). Reproductive outcome after laparoscopic myomectomy in infertile women. *J Reprod Med* **45**: 23–30.

57. Miller CE, Johnston M & Rundell M (1996). Laparoscopic myomectomy in the infertile woman. *Am Assoc Gynecol Laparosc* **3**: 525–32.

58. Rossetti A, Sizzi O, Soranna L, Mancuso S, Lanzone A (2001). Fertility outcome: long-term results after laparoscopic myomectomy. *Gynecol Endocrinol* **15**: 129–34.

6

Hysteroscopic myomectomy

Amelie Gervaise and Herve Fernandez

Hopital Antoine Beclere, Clamart, France

Operative hysteroscopy has modified the surgical approach to benign uterine lesions. Lesions that previously required a laparotomy can now be treated by hysteroscopy. Neuwirth & Amin[1] first described hysteroscopic resection of submucous myoma. This hysteroscopic management has reduced morbidity, duration of hospitalization and costs while attaining a success rate ranging from 67% to 98% for bleeding[2-6] and 21% to 60% for infertility.[7-14]

Classification of submucous myoma

Myoma can be divided into three groups according to the location of the largest part of the myoma.
- Subserous myoma: located on the peritoneal surface of the uterus.
- Intramural myoma: in the myometrium.
- Submucous myoma: myoma protruding into the uterine cavity.

Only submucous myoma can be treated by operative hysteroscopy.

The European Society for Human Reproduction and Embryology (ESHRE) classification of submucous myoma

There are three types of submucous myoma:
- Type 0: completely intracavitary (pedunculated myoma).
- Type 1: largest diameter in the uterine cavity.
- Type 2: largest diameter in the myometrium.

Type 0 and 1, and some type 2 myomas are accessible by hysteroscopy.

Contraindications of hysteroscopic myomectomy

The contraindications to operative hysteroscopy are contraindications to anesthesia, genital infections, pregnancy, and multiple myomas requiring myomectomy by laparotomy.

Preoperative preparation

Ultrasound

Abdominal and transvaginal ultrasound of the pelvis can determine the size and type of submucous myoma. For type 2 myoma, ultrasound allows measurement of the distance between the external margin of the myoma and the uterine serosa. This is important in order to assess the risk of uterine perforation during surgery.

Sonohysterography
This is a double contrast ultrasound with saline injected into the uterine cavity.

Diagnostic hysteroscopy

If the ultrasound results are unclear, diagnostic hysteroscopy will confirm whether the myoma is submucosal. It determines the number, size, type, and site.

Magnetic resonance imaging (MRI)

MRI is the most accurate tool to assess myoma. The site, position, number, and size of the myoma can be characterized. Moreover, it distinguishes myoma from adenomyosis, to a certain extent leiomyosarcoma and adnexal masses. MRI, however is costly.

Preoperative counseling

Before conducting hysteroscopic myomectomy, the patient must be informed about the:
- possible complications of uterine perforation, endometritis, and electrolytes imbalance;
- possibility that two separate interventions may be required for complete resection, especially for type 2 myoma or myoma of >4 cm in diameter;
- possibility that surgery may fail, necessitating a hysterectomy (very rare).

Preoperative medical treatment

The effects of gonadotropin-releasing hormone (GnRH) agonists on myoma and the endometrium are well documented. Gonadotropin-releasing hormone analog (GnRHa) decreases the myoma size, and induces an atrophic endometrium leading to a better visualization.[15,16] The smaller myoma and the decrease in vascularization leads to an easier procedure and less bleeding. The duration of preoperative treatment with GnRHa is usually two months.

In menopausal women with cervical stenosis, local or systemic estrogen therapy may be prescribed for two to three weeks to facilitate cervical dilatation. Cervical dilatation especially in nulligravid and menopausal women can be facilitated by administration of misoprostol (two tablets, intravaginally, two hours before surgery).

Set-up

Patient

- General or regional/local anesthesia (epidural or spinal).
- Dorsal recumbent (flat) position.
- Perineal and cervicovaginal disinfection.
- Antibiotic prophylaxis administered with induction of anesthesia to avoid the risk of endometritis.

Equipment

- Camera and monitor.
- Equipment to administer and monitor the distension media. For constant uterine distention, the pressure is continuously provided by irrigation and suction pumps.
- Standard tubings.
- Distension medium: glycine (1.5% solution packaged in 3-l plastic bags) is used for operative hysteroscopy with monopolar energy. Saline is used with bipolar energy.
- Light source.
- High-frequency power generator.
- Monopolar electrosurgical resection uses high-frequency current (>300 000 Hz).
- With bipolar current, the distention medium is saline (which reduces the risks of metabolic complications) and the instrument channel has a smaller diameter (which simplifies the dilatation). There are two settings, for vaporization and for desiccation. The maximum power used by the generator is 200 W.

Instrumentation

Standard instruments

- Bivalve speculum.
- Pozzi or Museux–Palmer forceps.
- Dilators: Hegar's dilators: 1 to 10 mm (increasing diameter from 0.5 or 1 mm).

- Hysterometer.
- Rigid hysteroscope: 2.7 mm to 4 mm in diameter; the usual angle for operative hysteroscopy is 12°.

For operative hysteroscopy with monopolar energy

- Resectoscope (7–9 mm), with internal (for irrigation) and external sheaths (for lavage).
- Surgical grip, either passive (electrode retracted) or active (electrode extended).
- 4-mm resection electrodes with a 90° 2 mm resection loop, 7–9 mm.

For operative hysteroscopy with bipolar energy

- 5–9 mm double-current sheath.
- Electrodes with a 24 French 90° resection loop, or a 5 French tip.

System settings

Monopolar system

The irrigation-suction pump must be pre-set to maintain a constant intrauterine pressure of ≤100 mm Hg, a flow-rate of 250 ml/s and a suction of 0.2 bar. Ideally, the operation should not last longer than 45 minutes. Although it is preferable not to use more than 6 l of glycine, the fluid deficit should not be over 500–1000 ml. The inflow and outflow of the distention fluid must be continuously checked. Surgery should be stopped if the fluid deficit is 1000 ml. In the case of a large fluid deficit or long surgery, serum electrolytes should be measured.

Bipolar system

This is a newer electrosurgical system. The safety and efficacy of this bipolar system appear equivalent to those of the monopolar technique. The diameter of the instrument channel remains the same for the new 24 French resection loops and is smaller for the 5 French bipolar tips. Instead of glycine, the distending medium is saline. The use

of saline decreases the risks of metabolic complications. The resection technique with 24-French electrodes and the length of surgery are similar to the standard hysteroscopic resection with monopolar electrode.

Besides the reduced risk of electrolyte imbalance, this system allows vaporization of myoma of < 2 cm. Absence of tissue debris with vaporization maintains the visualization and facilitates the operation.

Technique

Patient placement

Pelvic examination is first performed to assess the position of the uterus. A bivalve speculum is inserted, and the cervix is grasped with two Pozzi or Museux–Palmer forceps, placed at 3 o'clock and 9 o'clock, to move the uterus into an intermediate position. The surgery begins with a diagnostic hysteroscopy. The cervix is then dilated with Hegar's dilators, up to 10 mm.

Introduction of the resectoscope

The scope, hysteroscope and electrodes are assembled. It is important to purge the tubings from air bubbles. The resectoscope is introduced under hysteroscopic control. Hysteroscopic resection is performed using a cutting current.

Myoma resection

Pedunculated myoma
For type-0 pedunculated myoma <2 cm, the base of the myoma is resected at the level of the endometrium. The myoma is extracted with the loop (without current) or a blunt curette.

Type 0 myoma >2 cm is resected progressively from the surface of the myoma towards the endometrium.

Types 1 and 2 myomas
For types 1 and 2 myomas, resection is started from the intracavitary portion until the border

between the intramural portion of the myoma and myometrium (pink, less firm, and easily bleeds) is seen. Several methods can be used to stimulate extrusion of the intramural part into the uterine cavity including massage of the myoma with the loop, hydromassage by turning the on-off valve of the suction line repeatedly, and simultaneous injection of oxytocin (10 IU intravenously).

Difficult cases

In certain situations (myoma >4 cm, poor visualization, technical problems, surgical time >45 minutes or glycine deficit >500–1000 ml), the operator should discontinue the procedure. For submucous myoma located inside the uterine horn, extreme care is required to prevent injury to the tubal ostium or perforating the uterus.

Laser

Using a non-contact technique, the pedicle or the base of the myoma can be vaporized with 100 Watts of YAG laser. Myolysis can also be done by drilling the myoma with laser.

Postoperative management

Hysteroscopy is performed as an outpatient procedure. Systematic analgesia is not needed. A follow-up diagnostic hysteroscopy in two months may be needed in infertile women. This is to detect and treat a possible postoperative synechiae after myoma resection (10% of cases). The relatively fresh and fine synechiae can be easily removed using the beveled tip of the hysteroscope.

Complications

Mechanical complications

Most uterine perforations are encountered during cervical dilatation. It tends to occur in women with cervical stenosis, nulliparous or menopausal women and in those with acute retroverted or anteverted uterus. Depending on the size of the perforation, the procedure must be stopped and the patient is rescheduled two to three months later. Perforation during resection is less common, but more serious. Injury to the intestine, bladder, or large vessel can occur. Cervical tear and creation of a false passage are other possible complications during difficult dilatation. In these cases, a laparoscopy is indicated.

Infection

Post-hysteroscopic endometritis occurs in 1–5% of cases. We recommend prophylactic intraoperative antibiotics.[17]

Bleeding

Inserting a Foley catheter into the uterine cavity and inflating its balloon with 30 ml of saline can manage severe bleeding following a hysteroscopic myoma resection. The catheter can be removed in a few hours.

Metabolic complications

Operative hysteroscopy with monopolar energy

Glycine overload can cause electrolyte imbalance (hyponatremia, hypoproteinemia, and low hematocrit). Clinically, patients will complain of nausea, vomiting, headache, and confusion on awakening. Pulmonary and brain edema can occur in serious cases.

Operative hysteroscopy with bipolar energy

While fluid overload is possible with saline, its effects are less serious than those of glycine.

Gas embolisms

Embolisms can occur from gas produced by the electrosurgery or from room air. The risk of embolism from gas produced by bipolar electrosurgery is extremely low. Air embolism is more dangerous. The surgeons and the anesthetist should be aware about this potential complication and must know how to manage it.

Table 6.1. Menometrorrhagia and hysteroscopic treatment of submucous myoma (main series)

Authors	n	Size (cm)	Site SM-IP	Preop. LHRHa (A) Danazol (D)	Technique	Clinical success/ anatomic success (%)	Recurrence (%)	Follow up (months)	Repeat surgery (%)
Baggish et al.[2]	23	3	IP	D	Laser	80	?	?	?
Barbot & Parent[3]	825	1–6	SM + IP	A if > 4 cm	Laser	90/82.3	4.9	8–84	5
Corson & Brooks[18]	92	NA	NA	A or D	Resection	81/?	12	8–17	17.4
Cravello et al.[4]	239	0.5–6	SM + IP	A if > 4 cm	Resection	81/61.7	11.2	30 (6–67)	16.3
Derman et al.[19]	108	NA	NA	None	Resection	76/?	24.5	53	15.9
Donnez et al.[20]	376	<5	SM + IP	A if >4 cm or D	Laser	94/94	6.2	24	?
Hallez[5]	274	1–6.5	SM + IP	None	Resection	76.5/76.5	1.9	60	5.8
Loffer[21]	43	>1.5	SM	A or D	Resection	93/?	0 (at 1 year)	12–48	28.8
Mergui[22]	111	1–5	SM + IP	A	Resection	80/64.8	0	11	14.1
Vallee[23]	52	3.2 (1–9.5)	NA	A	Scissors	80/?	8	>3	?
Wamsteker[6]	51	NA	SM + IP	None	Resection	94/90	6	20 (10–34)	27.4
Fernandez et al.[24]	200	3 (1–7)	SM + IP	A if > 4 cm	Resection	74	16.50	33	13.60

NA: not applicable.

SM: sub mucous (type 0).

IP: interstitial (type 1 or 2).

Preop. LHRHa: preoperative luteinizing hormone releasing hormone analog.

Table 6.2. Fertility after hysteroscopic myomectomy

Authors	Number of patients	Pregnancies	Pregnancy rate (%)	Delivery rate (%)
Goldenberg et al.[25]	15	7	47	40
Donnez et al.[20]	24	16	67	67
Valle[23]	16	10	62	50
Corson & Brooks[18]	13	10	77	61
Giatras et al.[26]	41	25	61	49
Varasteh et al.[14]	36	19	53	36
Vercellini et al.[27]	40	15	37	32
Fernandez et al.[24]	59	16	27	10

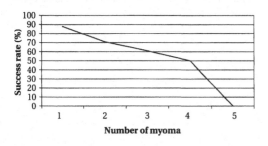

Figure 6.1. Success rate of hysteroscopic myomectomy as a function of the number of myoma.

Prevention of air and gas embolisms:
- Purge the tubing before beginning the procedure.
- In the case of cervical incompetence, close the external os with Pozzi forceps.
- Use a Y-tubing to reduce the risk of air entry when the fluid bag is changed.
- Avoid repeated insertion and removal of the hysteroscope to diminish any "piston" effect.
- Avoid touching the venous plexus.

Results

The results of hysteroscopic myomectomy are depicted in Table 6.1.[2–6,18–24] It shows that hystero-scopic myomectomy is an effective procedure. Poor results are related to the size of the myoma (>5 cm) or the percentage of the intramural portion (>50%). Preoperative treatment with GnRHa may be helpful. Success also depends on the number of myoma[24] (Figure 6.1). Table 6.2 shows that the effects of hysteroscopic myomectomy on fertility.[14,18,20,23–27]

REFERENCES

1. Neuwirth RS & Amin HK (1976). Excision of submucus with hysteroscopic control. *Am J Obstet Gynecol* **126**: 95–9.
2. Baggish MS, Sze EHM & Morgan G (1989). Hysteroscopic treatment of symptomatic submucous myomata uterine with the ND YAG Laser. *J Gynecol Surg* **15**: 27–30.
3. Barbot J & Parent B (1994). Echecs et/ou récidives après myomectomie par voie hystéroscopique. In *Les fibromes utérins. Dubuisson JB, ed*; pp. 67–75. Paris: Editions Arnette.
4. Cravello L, D'Ercole C, Boubli L & Blanc B (1995). Hysteroscopic treatment of uterine fibroids. *J Gynecol Surg* **11**: 227–32.
5. Hallez JP (1995). Single-stage total hysteroscopic myomectomies: indications, techniques and results. *Fertil Steril* **63**: 703–8.
6. Wamsteker K, Emanuel MH & De Kruif JH (1993). Transcervical hysteroscopic resection of submucous fibroids for abnormal uterine bleeding: results regarding the degree of intramural extension. *Obstet Gynecol* **82**: 736–40.
7. Seoud MA, Patterson R, Muasher SJ & Coddington CC (1992). Effects of myomas or prior myomectomy on in vitro fertilization performance. *J Assist Reprod Genet* **9**: 217–21.
8. Narayan R, Rajat AQ & Goswamy K (1994). Treatment of submucous fibroids and outcome of assisted conception. *J Am Assoc Gynecol Laparosc* **1**: 307–11.
9. Ramzi AM, Saltar M, Amin Y, Mansour RT, Serour GI & Aboulgher MA (1998). Uterine myomata and outcome of assisted reproduction. *Hum Reprod* **13**: 198–202.
10. Stovall TG (1994). The American College of Obstetricians and Gynecologists: Uterine leiomyomata. *ACOG-Technical Bulletin* **192**: 1–9.
11. Eldar-Geva T, Meagher S, Healy DL, MacLachlan V, Breheny S & Wood C (1998). Effects of intramural, subserosal and submucosal uterine fibroids on the outcome of assisted reproductive technology treatment. *Fertil Steril.* **70**: 687–91.
12. Bulletti C, De Ziegler D, Polli V & Flamigni C (1999). The role of leiomyomas in infertility. *J Am Assoc Gynecol Laparosc* **6**: 441–5.

13. Bernard G, Darai E, Poncelet C, Benifla JL & Madelenat P (2000). Fertility after hysteroscopic myomectomy: effect of intramural fibroids. *Eur J Obstet Gynecol Reprod Biol* **1**: 85–90.

14. Verasteh NN, Neuwirth RS, Levin B & Keltz MD (1999). Pregnancy rates after hysteroscopic polypectomy and myomectomy in infertile women. *Obtstet Gynecol* **94**(2): 168–71.

15. Friedman MR, Berbier RL & Benacerraf BR (1987). Treatment of leiomyomata with intranasal or subcutaneous leuprolide, a Gn-Rh agonist. *Fertil Steril* **48**: 560–9.

16. Lawrence AS, Healy DL, Hill D & Paterson PJ (1991). Management of submucous uterine fibroid with buserelin gemeprost and hysteroscopic resection. *Med J Aus.* **154**: 280–2.

17. McCausland V, Fields A & Townsend E (1993). Tuboovarian abscesses after operative hysteroscopy. *J Reprod Med* **38**: 198–200.

18. Corson SL & Brooks PG (1991). Resectoscopic myomectomy. *Fertil Steril* **55**: 1041–4.

19. Derman SG, Rehenstrom J & Neuwith RS (1991). The long term effectiveness of hysteroscopic treatment of menorrhagia and leiomyomas. *Obstet Gynecol* **77**: 591–4.

20. Donnez J, Gilklerot S, Bourgonjon D, Clerckx F & Nisolle M (1990). Neodymium: YAG laser hysteroscopy in large submucous fibroids. *Fertil Steril* **54**: 999–1003.

21. Loffer FD (1990). Removal of large symptomatic intrauterine growths by the hysteroscopic resectoscope. *Obstet Gynecol* **76**: 836–40.

22. Mergui JL, Renolleau C & Salat-Baroux J (1993). Hystéroscopie opératoire et fibromes. *Gynécologie* **1**: 325–37.

23. Valle RF (1990). Hysteroscopic removal of submucous leiomyomatas. *J Gynecol Surg* **6**: 89–96.

24. Fernandez H, Sefrioui O, Virelizier C, Gervaise A, Gomel V & Frydman R (2001). Hysteroscopic resection of submucosal myomas in patients with infertility. *Human Reprod* **16**: 1489–92.

25. Goldenberg M, Siuvan E, Sharabi Z, Biuder D, Rabinovici J & Seidman DS (1995). Outcome of hysteroscopic resection of submucous myoma for infertility. *Fertil Steril* **64**: 714–16.

26. Giatras K, Berkeley AS, Noyes N, Licciardi F, Lolis D & Grifo JA (1996). Fertility after hysteroscopic resection of submucous myomas. *J Am Assoc Gynec Laparosc* **2**: 155–8.

27. Vercellini P, Zaina B, Yaylayan L, Pisacreta A, De Giorgi O & Crosignani P (1999). Hysteroscopic myomectomy: long term effects on menstrual pattern and fertility. *Obstet Gynecol* **94**: 341–7.

7

Myomas in pregnancy

L. April Gago and Michael P. Diamond

Wayne State University School of Medicine, Michigan, USA

Leiomyomas are the most common tumor in pregnancy, with a reported prevalence of 0.09% to 3.9%.[1–6] These percentages reflect a range that on the low end indicate findings of older studies that relied on physical examination and diagnosis at the time of laparotomy or cesarean section. The upper range comes from more recent studies that utilized ultrasound examination to prospectively diagnose myomas during pregnancy. Overall, the reported prevalence of leiomyomata in reproductive age women is 20–40% with the higher rates quoted for African American women, and those with a family history of myomas.[7] The incidence of myomas increases progressively from menarche to menopause, with rates of 50% reported at the time of autopsy.[8,9] A genetic predisposition for the development of myomas has been proposed, although specific responsible genes have not been identified.

Older studies used physical examination and surgical findings for the diagnosis of myomas in pregnancy. This biased their findings toward larger and symptomatic myomas. Using ultrasound, the diagnosis of myomas in pregnancy is 1.5 to 4 times higher than previously reported. In a retrospective study, Rice et al. noted that only 25% of myomas <5 cm in diameter were detected on physical examination, and only 50% of myomas >5 cm were diagnosed when compared to ultrasound.[10] It is clear that the use of routine ultrasound examinations increases the recognition of myomas in pregnancy.[3,4,10]

Genetic origins of myomas

Myomas arise from a mutation in a single smooth muscle, myometrial cell. Townsend et al. first established this in their classic study, which identified individual myoma cells as identical by their glucose-6-phosphate electrophoretic type.[11] Spontaneous chromosome rearrangements are likely responsible for the initiation and progression of leiomyoma growth. Various cytogenetic abnormalities have been identified in these cell lines, but no single chromosomal defect has been found.

Most myomas have normal karyotypes. However, there are several consistent translocations and deletions involving chromosomes 14q24 and 7q22 that are associated with myomas. It appears that the deletions involving 7q22 may disable an unidentified tumor suppressor gene. Similarly, the activation of a specific oncogene such as *fos*, which is known to reside on 14q24, could be a mechanism for the initiation of myoma development. *Fos* is an appealing candidate as a major player in myoma formation, as estrogen stimulates its mRNA production. Additionally, the oncogene *met* has been localized in the chromosome region 7q31–32, and clonal rearrangements involving 7q31–32 in myoma specimens have been reported.[12] The absence of clonal rearrangements noted in most leiomyoma specimens may possibly be explained by the inability of routine cytogenetic techniques to detect low levels of mosaicism and point mutations. Altering these observations may indicate the presence of normal cells that grow preferentially in culture.[11]

Once the neoplastic transformation has occurred, there are several agents known to stimulate myoma growth. Estrogen has been associated with the growth of uterine myomas, as noted by their increasing prevalence after menarche, regression at menopause, and after GnRH analog therapy. Serum estradiol concentrations are not higher in women with myomas,[13] but more estrogen receptors in myomatous tissue have been reported.[14] Also, there is a local increase in estrogen bioactivity as a result of a lower conversion rate of estradiol to estrone in leiomyomata than in myometrium.[15] These findings are supported by the reports of endometrial hyperplasia at the margins of submucous myomas.[16] Increasing evidence suggests that the mitogenic effects of estrogen are mediated by several growth factors such as growth hormone, insulin-like growth factors I and II, epidermal growth factor, and transforming growth factor-β (TGF-β).[17–19] TGF-β has been localized to 14q23–24, also a common region for aberrations in myomas, and appears to be involved in a variety of neoplastic processes as a tumor suppressor.[20]

Myomas and infertility

The clinical impact of myomas is large, as they contribute to a variety of conditions including infertility, recurrent pregnancy loss, various complications of pregnancy, as well as menorrhagia and dysmenorrhea. Approximately 40% of women with multiple myomas have a history of infertility. In contrast, 5% of infertile patients have myomas, with myomas as the only cause in 2–3%.[8]

Mechanisms by which myomas cause infertility may include: (1) disruption of the endometrial contour that interferes with implantation; (2) implantation directly over a myoma may result in insufficient blood supply for proper placentation; (3) discordant endometrial growth and maturation may hinder natural implantation; (4) changes in local paracrine factors may create an inhospitable milieu for sperm and/or embryos; (5) anatomic distortion caused by myomas may reduce access to the cervix by sperm, and interferes with sperm transport; (6) enlarged uterine cavity increases the distance sperm must travel; (7) altered uterine contractility may impede sperm and embryo transport; and (8) uterine myoma may cause tubal narrowing.[7,8,21]

The actual impact of myomas and the benefit of myomectomy on infertility are still unclear. Distortions of endometrial cavity by submucous and intramural myomas have been consistently shown to decrease fertility.[22,23] The results of studies of women with myomas that do not distort the cavity are mixed. In a prospective study of 91 cycles of assisted reproductive technology (ART) in women with myomas and no cavity distortion, the pregnancy rate was significantly lower in the myoma group (37.4% vs 52.7%).[24] Also, it appears that intramural myomas may have some negative impact on fertility when examined separately from subserosal tumors. Eldar-Geva et al. specifically looked at intramural myomas versus subserosal versus controls and found pregnancy rates of 16.4%, 34.1%, and 30.1% respectively.[25]

Previous works had combined intramural and subserosal tumors with inconsistent conclusions on the effect on fertility. The low rate (5.5%) of subserosal tumors included in one study may account for these discrepancies.[24] It appears that the closer the myoma is to the endometrial cavity, the higher the negative impact is on fertility. Submucous myoma are the most detrimental, followed by intramural, with subserosal myoma having little effect.

Myomectomy as a fertility therapy is fraught with controversy. The literature tends to support an increased conception rate in the first year after a myomectomy.[10,26–29] All of these studies are inherently confounded by many factors, but show a consistent decrease in miscarriage rates after removal of intracavitary lesions. The gains in fertility potential must be balanced against potential adverse effects including post-myomectomy adhesions, disruption of endometrium and synechiae formation, and tubal damage. Proper surgical techniques including the utilization of hysteroscopic approach when feasible can minimize these concerns.[21] The use of adhesion barriers and GnRH analogs may also be helpful. The recurrence of myomas after myomectomy is $\geq 25\%$. However, generally there is a sufficient delay to allow conception to occur.[26]

Myomas and pregnancy loss

Myomas have been associated with miscarriages and recurrent pregnancy loss.[16,30–32] Lev-Toaff et al. found that myomas located in the uterine corpus confer a greater risk of spontaneous abortion than those located elsewhere.[32] The miscarriage rate of women with a single myoma is 7%, and those with multiple myomas is 15%.[6] However, Muram et al. did not find an increased rate of miscarriage in their ultrasound study.[28]

Myomectomy decreases the miscarriage rates. In a review of 1941 cases, the loss rates were reduced from 41% before surgery to 19% after myomectomy.[8] Li et al. found a reduction from 60% to 24% after myomectomy using microsurgical techniques.[31] Similar to infertility, myoma-related pregnancy loss has been associated with thin, poorly decidualized endometrium, insufficient blood supply, increased uterine contractility, or inflammatory processes of the endometrium secondary to myoma degeneration. All of these could potentially compromise placental development and/or placentation, resulting in pregnancy failure.

Myoma behavior in pregnancy

Several prospective studies utilizing ultrasound surveillance have described the natural history of leiomyoma in pregnancy. One of the landmark papers was published by Muram et al. in 1980 and their ultrasound characterization of myomas have become known as the Muram criteria.[28] They distinguished myomas ultrasonographically by identification of a mass that fulfilled the following criteria: (1) greater than 3 cm in diameter; (2) relatively spherical; (3) distortion of the myometrial contour by the mass

either externally or by impingement on the gestational sac; and (4) different acoustical structure of the mass than the myometrium. Additional criteria that fulfilled the first four include; (1) a speckled pattern of internal echoes, increasing in density with increased ultrasound sensitivity; and (2) no enhancement of echoes behind the mass suggesting a cystic nature.

Using color Doppler imaging, Kessler et al. added further characterization of myoma.[33] In myoma, distortion and splaying of blood vessels around the periphery of the uterine mass is demonstrated. In contrast, crowding of blood vessels centrally is seen in uterine contraction. Uterine contractions are also transient. Accordingly, rescanning the mass after 30 minutes assists in diagnosis. Lev-Toaff et al. described ultrasound characteristics of myomas as patterns of hypoechoic, heterogeneous masses, frequently having an echogenic rim.[32]

The development of cystic spaces and increased heterogeneity during the pregnancy is not uncommonly found. Cystic changes are found in 23% of myomas in the first trimester and in 32% in the second trimester of gestation. Interestingly, 70% of patients with changes in the echotexture of the uterine mass developed abdominal pain versus 11.7% of those without such changes. These echotexture changes were not associated with significant changes in the dimensions of the myomas. Based on their findings in 113 pregnancies, the authors felt that the development of an echogenic rim was a final ultrasonic pattern in myoma evolution.[33]

Contrary to widespread beliefs, in most cases there is no significant or steady growth of myomas during pregnancy. In general, myoma growth occurs mainly in the first trimester and does not continue beyond it. Four longitudinal ultrasound studies have revealed these patterns. In the Muram et al. study, there was no significant change in the myoma size (defined as >10% change) in 38 of 41 women.[28] In two women, the myoma size increased by 20–25% and in another, the size decreased by 20%. In a larger longitudinal study, the size of myoma in pregnancy did not change much.[32] In the first trimester, the myomas either remained unchanged or increased in size. In the second trimester, small myomas increased while large myomas decreased in size. In the third trimester, all myomas diminished in size.

In another prospective study, Strobelt et al. found that 15% of myomas increased in size (defined as > 10% increase), and 85% remained stable or decreased during the second and third trimester, with 62% disappearing completely.[4] Seventy-five percent of myomas of < 5 cm were not visualized at follow-up scan. A smaller study that followed 32 myomas in 29 pregnancies found that 59% remained unchanged in size, 22% increased greater than 10% in size, but none by more than 25%, and 19% decreased in size. Thirteen of these patients had postpartum scans and only five myomas were visualized, three decreased in size and two increased.[34] Another study also found no changes in myoma during pregnancy.[27] In this study, they noted that 69% of women had a single myoma, 19% had two and 12% had three or more. As the number of myomas increased, their size tended to decrease. The mean reported volume increase of myomas in pregnancy is around 12%; none have noted growth greater than 25%.[32,34]

Myomatous degeneration

The most common complication associated with myomas in pregnancy is degeneration. This is often referred to as "red degeneration, carneous degeneration or hemorrhagic infarction." The degeneration is thought to be the consequence of necrosis of the myoma as the growth of the uterus creates a rotation of the myoma relative to its blood supply with ensuing torsion and infarction. It has also been suggested that progesterone may induce this degenerative process. The clinical findings of this syndrome include pain over the myoma, leukocytosis, nausea and vomiting, and mild pyrexia. However, recent series have described the more common presentation as simply localized pain over the myoma with cystic and heterogeneous patterns on ultrasound.[2–4,6,35] The incidence of myoma degeneration in pregnancy is 10–25%.[2,3,6,10]

Hasan et al. reported that the incidence of degenerative symptoms in pregnancy was 10%.[2] Four of their patients underwent exploratory laparotomy for preoperative diagnosis of torsion. In a retrospective chart review of 123 492 cases, Burton et al. found 106 deliveries complicated by myomas.[5] Fourteen or 0.01% required laparotomy. Among these, five patients were found to have myomas, judged too large to be removed safely. These included large myomas ($8 \times 10 \times 7$ cm; 12×18 cm; 10×14 cm), and those with stalks >5 cm in diameter. Six women underwent myomectomy during pregnancy due to severe pain. All had stalks 2–5 cm in diameter. Five of them subsequently had term deliveries. Another had an aborting cervical myoma, subsequently had chorioamnionitis, fetal death at 20 weeks, and hysterectomy. Another patient required laparotomy at postpartum period for an infected pedunculated myoma. Thirteen patients in this review had an incidental myomectomy at the time of cesarean delivery. Two-thirds were asymptomatic during pregnancy. Bleeding requiring transfusion complicated one case. Degenerative changes were found in 70% of the specimens. In addition to surgical complications, 25% of these patients required hospitalization for abdominal pain, and 13% experienced preterm labor.

In a study of 492 pregnant women who had myoma, 62 (13%) women experienced pelvic pain.[6] On ultrasound, 82 women were found to have cystic spaces and heterogeneous echo patterns on their myoma. The authors found a correlation between myoma size of >200 cm^3 and the painful degeneration syndrome. Thirty-two patients were managed surgically; 13 had myomectomies during pregnancy; 9 had myomectomy at the time of cesarean section with three of these requiring hysterectomy; and an additional 10 required hysterectomy at the time of delivery for hemorrhage. The indications of myomectomy in pregnancy were myoma degeneration, intractable pain or fever. All myomas were subserous or pedunculated, and larger than 100 cm^3. All of these antepartum myomectomies were performed after 26 weeks of gestation and resulted in deliveries more than seven weeks after the procedure. Compared to women without myoma (0.4%), postpartum sepsis occurred in 4% of the cases.[6]

Katz et al. reviewed the records of 6005 women with ultrasound diagnosis and found 121 myomatous pregnancies (2%). There were 31 admissions among 25 patients for myoma related pain.[3] The pain occurred in the second and early third trimester with an average gestational age of 20.4 weeks (10–34 weeks). The overall pregnancy outcome was good. For pain related degeneration, the authors recommended ibuprofen 600–800 mg orally every six hours. Because of the potential risk of premature closure of the ductus arteriosus, neonatal pulmonary hypertension, and potential platelet dysfunction, ibuprofen should not be administered after 34 weeks of gestation.

The average hospital stays for patients treated with ibuprofen was 2.1 days versus 3.8 days for those treated with narcotics.[3] Dildy et al. used indomethacin 25 mg orally every six hours in seven cases of degenerating myomas that had failed prior treatment with tocolytics and narcotics.[35] All had relief of symptoms within 48 hours. Five of the seven had term deliveries without complication. Two delivered prematurely at 21 and 22 weeks gestation.

Preterm labor and premature rupture of membranes, and abruption

Myomas have been inconsistently associated with vaginal bleeding, preterm onset of labor (POL), and preterm premature rupture of membranes (PPROM).[1,2,4,5,33,34] Rice et al. found an increase in POL from 20% for myomas ranging from 3 cm to 4.9 cm in size to 28% for those >5 cm.[10] No increase rate of POL was found in myomas <3 cm.[4] However, others could not confirm their findings.[6,39] The possible relationship between PPROM, POL and myomas are not well understood. However, it seems that there is a link between retroplacental myomas, POL, PPROM, and vaginal bleeding in pregnancy.[28]

The rate of abruption is increased in the presence of myoma.[1,6,10] In a population based, retrospective study, women with myomas were found to have a nearly twofold increased risk of abruption and PPROM.[1] Rice et al. found that myomas greater than 3 cm were associated with both POL and abruptio placentae.[10] They also noted a marked increased risk of abruption with retroplacental myomas, 57% versus 2.5% for those without retroplacental myomas.

The perinatal mortality rate for abruptions in pregnancies with retroplacental myomas was 50%, while the reported fetal death rate secondary to abruption in the general population is 0.2%. Even when other confounding variables were taken into account, this difference persisted. Overall, any myoma increased the abruption rate to 10.8% compared to a normal baseline of 1.1%.[10]

Lev-Toaff et al. found no relationship between placental and myoma location.[32] Coronado et al. found an almost fourfold increase in the rate of abruption in their retrospective chart review of 2065 pregnancies.[1] However, not all of their patients had ultrasound. In another retrospective chart review, Exacoustos et al. found a significantly increased risk of abruption in patients with myomas compared to controls, 7.5% versus 0.9%.[6] Again, these findings persisted, even when confounding factors such as hypertension were examined. Davis et al. however, in a prospective study of 85 pregnancies, found no increase in the rate of abruption, despite the finding of retroplacental myomas in 58% of the patients.[27] Predictably, 77% of women with two myomas had a retroplacental myoma and 90% of those with three or more myomas had this purported risk factor. Others have also not found an increase in the rate of abruption.[2,34]

Intrauterine fetal growth

Altered placental perfusion related to retroplacental myomas has been hypothesized to place the fetus at risk for intrauterine growth restriction. However, the existing literature has not substantiated these concerns.[6,10,27,32] Others have found lower birth weights, but this may be due to earlier delivery.[6] There have been numerous case reports of fetal malformations secondary to large submucosal myomas, including torticollis with deformation of the fetal head, as well as limb and postural deformities.[29,36,37]

Malpresentation

Malpresentation as a consequence of uterine deformity by the myoma has been reported. Coronado et al. found a fourfold increased risk of malpresentation in pregnancies complicated by myomas compared to controls.[1] Others reported that these increases were found only with retroplacental myoma or with myoma in the lower uterine segment.[10,32]

Cesarean section

The literature regarding the increased rate of Cesarean section in patients with myomas is quite consistent.[1-3,10,27,32] However, there are many confounding factors. Retrospective reviews rely on documentation of myomas in the chart, and specifically, rely heavily on the findings at the time of Cesarean section.[1-3,10] The trend of increased Cesarean sections in women with myomas persists in the prospective studies, but the magnitude of the increased risk is smaller.[6,27,32] The confounding factors are advanced maternal age and obstetrician's attitude. There is a tendency to perform a primary Cesarean section or to be more prone to Cesarean section due to the fears of complications or eventual arrest of labor. Overlapping risk factors include fetal malpresentation, dysfunctional labor, and abruption. Previous myomectomy also plays a role in higher cesarean deliveries as recurrence of myomas after myomectomy is about 25%.[26]

Management of myomas in pregnancy

Myomas are found in approximately 2% of pregnancies, with 10–30% of them having complications.[2,3,32] We recommend serial ultrasound examination for the documentation of echotexture changes in size, or the rare complications of fetal deformity.[10,28,32,36,37] There is some evidence that myomas >3 cm in size, and retroplacental myomas predispose to a higher risk of abruption, POL, and PPROM.[1,6,10,28] The most common complication is abdominal pain due to myoma degeneration. This occurs in 10–25% of cases and most often in the second and early third trimester.[2,3,6,10] Management of myomatous degeneration in pregnancy with nonsteroidal

anti-inflammatory agents is safe, effective, and appropriate prior to 34 weeks of gestation. If these fail, narcotics can be administered.

If medical management has failed, and the diagnosis is uncertain, exploratory laparotomy may be required. In the rare situation, myomectomy in pregnancy is indicated. Prior to performing myomectomy, one should consider gestational age, size and position of the myoma, and extent of degeneration. Excision of intramural and submucous myomas may be associated with bleeding and spontaneous abortion.

Myomectomy at the time of Cesarean section should be judiciously performed. There is a risk of hemorrhage and hysterectomy. Necrotic myomas are the perfect medium for anaerobic infection. The infection could be severe and resistant to antibiotics. In one study, the incidence of myoma-related postpartum sepsis is 4% compared to a 0.4% rate in those without myomas.[6] Aggressive use of antibiotics with good anaerobic coverage in patients with myomas and postpartum endomyometritis is prudent. Cesarean section appears to be significantly higher in patients with myomas,[1-3,10,27,32] and they should be counseled as such. Dysfunctional labor, malpresentation, and abruption are the major indications that have been elucidated.[1,10,32] Existing studies suggest that the rate of myoma-related complications of pregnancy is 10–30%.[2,4,32] Nonetheless, most of these are transient with good maternal and neonatal outcomes. Women with myomas should be educated about potential risks, but need not be discouraged to conceive.

Summary

Myomas are found in 0.9–3.9% of pregnancies.[1-6] Their prevalence has been increasing as women proceed through the reproductive years. A genetic predisposition, including African American background, places some women at increased risk of developing myomas at a younger age. The specific chromosomal abnormalities have not yet been elucidated, but evidence suggests that tumor suppressor genes or oncogenes are involved.[12] Estrogen as a necessary cofactor in this process is supported by myoma growth predominately under estrogen dominant hormonal conditions.

It appears that myoma plays a role in infertility[22,23] and myomectomy has been shown to improve conception rates, especially when the lesions are submucosal and intramural.[7,8,21,25] A similar relationship has been shown with miscarriages.[4,8,29,31,32] Prospective ultrasound studies of myomas throughout pregnancy have shown that there is an increased growth of less than 25% mainly in the first trimester.[4,27,28,32,34] Myomatous degeneration is the most common complication of pregnancy, and results in abdominal pain, sometimes requiring hospitalization. Conservative management with nonsteroidal anti-inflammatory medications is generally successful. In the rare situation, surgical intervention in pregnancy is required. This is due to myoma degeneration, torsion, or deformation of the fetus.[5,36,38] Other complications of pregnancy that have been variably associated with myomas include POL and PPROM.[1,6,10,39] Abruption appears to be a more consistent risk of myomatous uteri, especially when the myomas are retroplacental.[2,7,10] Other risks are malpresentation and Cesarean section.[1-3,10,27,32]

The number of women conceiving during their advanced reproductive years, and even exceeding the usual reproductive years with assisted reproductive technologies, continues to increase. Because they are known to play a role in fertility, fecundity, and mode of delivery, myomas in pregnancy will remain an important subject for clinical and basic science review and study.

REFERENCES

1. Coronado GD, Marshall LM & Schwartz SM (2002). Complications in pregnancy, labor, and delivery with uterine leiomyomas: a population-based study. *Obstet Gyn* **95**(5): 764–9.

2. Hasan F., Arumugan K & Sivanesaratnam V (1990). Uterine leiomyomata in pregnancy. *Internat J Gynecol Obstet* **34**: 45–8.

3. Katz VL, Dotters DJ & Droegemueller W (1989). Complications of uterine leiomyomas in pregnancy. *Obstet Gynecol* **73**: 593.

4. Strobelt N, Ghidini A, Cavallone M, Pensabene I, Ceruti P & Vergani P (1994). Natural history of uterine leiomyomas in pregnancy. *J Ultrasound Med* **13**: 399–401.

5. Burton CA, Grimes DA & March CM (1989). Surgical management of leoiomyomata during pregnancy: *Obstet Gynecol* **74**: 707.

6. Exacoustos C & Rosati P (1993). Ultrasound diagnosis of uterine myomas and complications in pregnancy. *Obstet Gynecol* **82**: 97–101.

7. American Society for Reproductive Medicine (2001). *A Practice Committee Report: Myomas and Reproductive Function.* Birmingham, Alabama: American Society for Reproductive Medicine.

8. Buttram VC & Reiter RC (1981). Uterine leiomyomata: etiology, symptomatology, and management. *Fertil Steril* **36**: 433–45.

9. Rock JA & Thompson JD (1997). *TeLinde's Operative Gynecology*, 8th edn, p. 732. Philadelphia: Lippincott-Raven Publishers.

10. Rice JP, Kay HH & Mahony BS (1989). The clinical significance of uterine leiomyoma in pregnancy. *Am J Obstet Gynecol* **160**: 1212–6.

11. Townsend DE, Sparks RS, Baluda MC & McCelland G (1970). Unicellular histogenesis of uterine leiomyomas as determined by electrophoresis of glucose-6-phosphate dehydrogenase. *Am J Obstet Gynecol* **107**: 1168–74.

12. Rein MS, Friedman AJ, Barbierei RL, et al. (1991). Cytogenetic abnormalities in uterine leiomyomata. *Obstet Gynecol* **77**: 923–6.

13. Spellacy WN, LeMaire WJ, Buhi WC, Birk SA & Bradley BA (1972). Plasma growth hormone and estradiol levels in women with uterine myomas. *Obstet Gynecol* **40**: 829–34.

14. Wilson EA, Frank Y & Rees ED (1980). Estradiol and progesterone binding in uterine leiomyomata and in normal uterine tissues. *Obstet Gynecol* **55**: 20–4.

15. Pollow K, Sinnecker G, Boquoi E & Pollow B (1978). In vitro conversion of estradiol-17β into estrone in normal human myometrium and leiomyoma. *J Clin Chem Clin Biochem* **16**: 493–502.

16. Deligdish L & Loewenthal M (1970). Endometrial changes associated with myomata of the uterus. *J Clin Path* **23**: 676–80.

17. Adashi EY, Rock JA & Rosenwaks Z (1996). *Endocrinology, Surgery, and Technology.* Philadelphia: Lippincott-Raven Publishers.

18. Rein MS, Friedman AJ, Pandian MR, et al. (1990). The

secretion of insulin-like growth factors I and II by explant cultures of fibroids and myometrium from women treated with a gonadotropin-releasing hormone agonist. *Obstet Gynecol* **76**: 390–4.

19. Fayed YM, Tsibris JC, Langenberg PW & Robertson AL (1989). Human uterine leiomyoma cells: binding and growth responses to epidermal growth factor, platelet-derived growth factor, and insulin. *Lab Invest* **60**: 30–7.

20. Sporn MB & Robert AB (1989). Transforming growth factor-β: Multiple actions and potential applications. *JAMA* **262**: 938–41.

21. Rahul S & Seifer DB (2002). Do uterine myomas cause infertility? *Infert Reprod Med Clin N Am* **13**: 315–24.

22. Ramzy AM, Sattar M, Amin Y, Mansour RT, Serour GI & Aboulghar MA (1998). Uterine myomata and outcome of assisted reproduction. *Europ Soc Hum Reprod Embryol* **13**: 198–202.

23. Farhi J, Ashkenazi J, Feldberg D, Dicker D, Orvieto R & Ben Rafael Z (1995). Effect of uterine leiomyomata on the results of in-vitro fertilization treatment. *Hum Reprod* **10**: 2576–8.

24. Stovall DW, Parrish SB, Van Voorhis BJ, Hahn SJ, Sparks AET & Syrop CH (1998). Uterine leiomyomas reduce the efficacy of assisted reproduction cycles: results of a matched follow-up study. *Hum Reprod* **13**: 192–7.

25. Eldar-Geva T, Meagher S, Healy DL, MacLachlan V, et al. (1998). Effect of intramural, subserosal, and submucosal uterine fibroids on the outcome of assisted reproductive technology treatment. *Fertil Steril* **70**: 687–91.

26. Verkauf BS (1992). Myomectomy for fertility enhancement and preservation. *Fertil Steril* **58**: 1–15.

27. Davis JL, Ray-Mazumder S, Hobel CJ, Baley K & Sassoon D (1990). Uterine leiomyomas in pregnancy: a prospective study: *Obstet Gynecol* **75**: 41.

28. Muram D, Gillieson M & Walters JH (1980). Myomas of the uterus in pregnancy: ultrasonographic follow-up. *Am J Obstet Gynecol* **18**: 16–19.

29. Ouyang DW & Hill III JA (2002). Leiomyomas, pregnancy, and pregnancy loss. *Infert Reprod Med Clin N Am* **13**: 325–39.

30. Diamond MP & Polan ML (1989). Intrauterine synechiae and leiomyomas in the evaluation and treatment of repetitive spontaneous abortions. *Semin Reprod Endocrinol* **7**: 111–14.

31. Li TC, Mortimer R & Cooke ID (1999). Myomectomy: a retrospective study to examine reproductive performance before and after surgery. *Hum Reprod* **14**: 1735–40.

32. Lev-Toaff AS, Coleman BG, Arger PH, Minta MC, Arenson RL & Toaff ME (1987). Leiomyomas in pregnancy: sonographic study. *Radiology* **164**: 375–80.

33. Kessler A, Mitchell DG, Kuhlman K & Goldberg BB (1993). Myomas vs. contraction in pregnancy: Differentiation with color Doppler imaging. *J Clin Ultrasound* **21**: 241–4.

34. Aharoni A, Reiter A, Golan D, Paltiely Y & Sharf M (1988). Patterns of growth of uterine leiomyomas during pregnancy. A prospective longitudinal study. *Br J Obstet Gyn* **95**: 510–13.

35. Dildy GA, Moise KJ, Smith LG, Kirshon B & Carpenter RJ (1992). Indomethacin for the treatment of symptomatic uterine leiomyoma during pregnancy. *Am J Perinatol* **9**: 185–9.

36. Joo JG, Knovay J, Silhavy M & Papp Z (2001). Successful enucleation of a necrotizing fibroid causing oligohydramnios and fetal postural deformity in the 25th week of gestation. A case report. *J Reprod Med* **46**(10): 923–5.

37. Romero R, Chervenak FA, DeVore G, Tortora M & Hobbins JC (1981). Fetal head deformation and congenital torticollis associated with a uterine tumor. *Am J Obstet Gynecol* **141**(7): 839–40.

38. Winer-Muram HT, Muram D & Gillieson MS (1983). Uterine myomas in pregnancy. *Can Med Assoc J* **128**: 949–50.

39. Febo G, Tessarolo L, Leo L, Arduino S, Wierdis T & Lanza L (1997). Surgical management of leiomyomata in pregnancy. *Clin Exp Obst Gyn* **24**(2): 76–8.

8

Expectant and medical management of uterine fibroids

William W. Brown III and Charles C. Coddington III

Department of Obstetrics and Gynecology, Mail Code 0660, Colorado, USA

Expectant Management

The decision to treat a patient with an enlarged and symptomatic uterine fibroid is typically straightforward. However, the best approach in asymptomatic women with an enlarged uterus is not always clear. Uterine leiomyomata occur in the vast majority of women,[1] but the total prevalence is unknown. Of the total 600 000 hysterectomies performed each year, 20–30% are due to uterine fibroids[2] and some of these hysterectomies are done merely due to an enlarged uterus.

The initial diagnostic dilemma for the clinician when a patient presents with a large pelvic mass is to determine its origin. The reasons many gynecologists have not pursued expectant treatment and the rationale of this type of management will be discussed in this review.

Predictable growth of uterine fibroids

There are no data to support the concept that myomas will continue to grow. It is known, however, that fibroids will shrink after menopause. This is due to the decline in endogenous estrogen levels. Racial differences, body mass index (BMI) and parity are factors that affect the risk of developing clinically significant leiomyomas. Nevertheless, good information on the natural history of the disease is lacking.[3,4] One recent report suggests that some small myomas, if simply observed, will regress.[5]

Missed or delayed diagnosis of uterine sarcoma

The size of the uterus poorly predicts the likelihood of malignancy.[6] In a retrospective study,[7] 1332 women with enlarged uterine myoma were surgically treated. Three patients were found to have uterine sarcoma (one leiomyosarcoma and two endometrial stromal sarcoma), for a total incidence of 0.23%. This report confirmed the relative rarity of sarcoma of the uterus. More importantly, it also questions the notion that these malignant neoplasms tend to grow rapidly. Of those patients treated for fibroids, either upon abstraction of the hospital chart or review of the physician's office record, 371 were noted to have rapid growth of the uterus with an increase of at least six gestational weeks over the one year prior to surgery. Yet, only one of the 371 patients (0.27%) was found to have uterine sarcoma. Thus, accelerated or rapid growth of a presumed fibroid uterus, especially in a premenopausal woman, is no longer a reason to recommend a hysterectomy. In fact, the risk of sarcoma closely approaches the operative mortality rate for hysterectomy.[8,9]

Uterine sarcoma is more commonly seen in postmenopausal women, with the mean age at diagnosis of 54–63 years,[10] whereas the incidence of leiomyomata peaks at 40–44 years.[11] Unfortunately, current imaging techniques, such as ultrasonography or magnetic resonance imaging (MRI) do not predict these cancers with a high degree of diagnostic accuracy. Transcervical needle biopsy is a recently described technique that has a strong negative predictive value for distinguishing uterine sarcoma from leiomyoma.[12] Although, myomas and sarcomas may both produce similar signs and symptoms, there are clinical scenarios that should increase the physician's level of suspicion for an underlying malignancy. These include a worsening clinical course with continued uterine enlargement and/or bleeding while under treatment with leuprolide acetate,[13] and bleeding and pain in a postmenopausal patient with an enlarged uterus. Most patients with leiomyosarcomas present with abnormal bleeding.[14]

Inability to clinically evaluate the adnexa

The argument that hysterectomy is indicated in women with large uterine fibroids to facilitate adnexal examination is not evidence based. Today, high-resolution pelvic ultrasound and MRI can be helpful to evaluate the ovaries in the presence of uterine enlargement.

Pelvic examination is not a useful screening technique for asymptomatic ovarian malignancy.[4] In fact, the National Institutes of Health and National Cancer Institute Consensus Conference suggests that palpation of the adnexa is a poor means for detecting early ovarian cancer.[15] Seventy-five percent (75%) of ovarian cancers are already outside the confines of the ovary at the time of initial diagnosis,[16] and ovarian cancer diagnosed in the presence of uterine leiomyomata is not more apt to be an advanced stage of the disease. Accordingly, hysterectomy or myomectomy does not improve the likelihood of diagnosing early ovarian cancer.

Increased surgical risk and technical difficulty with a larger tumor bulk

Both hysterectomy and myomectomy are associated with a certain degree of morbidity and surgical risk. Due to the belief that operative morbidity paralleled uterine size, gynecologists often recommend surgical intervention when the fibroid uterus is greater than 12 gestational weeks. A larger uterus requires a larger incision and may be more difficult to remove, but there is no basis for predicting

the future behavior of leiomyomata in an individual patient.

Reiter et al. showed that in 93 women who underwent hysterectomy for uterine fibroids, the complication rate was not related to the size of the uterus.[17] This is in contrast with the findings of Hillis et al.[18] Their study had a larger sample size (466 patients). When the fibroid uterus was larger than 500 g, or about 14–18 weeks size, the patient suffered more blood transfusion, cuff cellulitis and other complications. In a smaller study, Stewart et al. demonstrated that a large, solitary myoma is more easily and completely removed than multiple leiomyomata.[19] Thus, smaller and multiple myomata have a higher level of recurrence. Clinically, there are not many women with a fibroid uterus larger than 18 weeks in size that are totally asymptomatic.

Reproductive performance

The effects of uterine leiomyomata on reproduction remain unclear. The impact of fibroids may be related to tubal occlusion due to the enlarging myoma, alteration in tubal function, distortion of the cervix in relation to the vaginal pool of semen, submucosal location inhibiting normal placental implantation, decreased oxytocinase activity and decreased uterine expansion resulting in preterm labor, decidual necrosis, or distortion of the uterine cavity. Studies have shown that in the absence of other infertility factors, myomectomy may improve conception rates.[20,21] Spontaneous abortion rates may also decrease.[22,23] However, the surgeon must weigh the risks and benefits of myomectomy against the occurrence of postoperative adhesions, the morbidity of the procedure, and the potential for fibroid recurrence, which may vary from 15% to 45%.[4]

The effects of fibroids on pregnancy outcome are less clear. Studies to date suggest that the Cesarean section rate is increased, but the data on the occurrence of abruptio placenta, low birth rate and premature rupture of membranes are conflicting.[24,25] It is clinically unfounded for the practitioner to recommend myomectomy for asymptomatic women desiring pregnancy with no history of infertility or recurrent pregnancy loss. It may be wise, however, to counsel the patient about the small risks of degeneration and pain in pregnancy.

Compromise of nearby pelvic organs

The prevalence of this condition has never been documented. Of greatest concern is ureteral obstruction, and this is more likely an issue in a very large, symmetrical fibroid uterus. An intravenous pyelogram or renal ultrasound can help in the management of these patients. Mild degrees of stable hydroureter and hydronephrosis in the presence of normal kidney function do not necessitate intervention.

Uterine growth and bleeding with hormone replacement therapy (HRT)

One report suggests that oral contraceptives do not enhance fibroid growth.[26] Whether hormone replacement therapy promotes the growth of the fibroid is unclear.[27] Women who experience vaginal bleeding or enlarging fibroid can be managed simply by discontinuation of their HRT. The etiology of the bleeding, however, has to be investigated.

In summary, there is no evidence to support prophylactic hysterectomy or myomectomy in the presence of asymptomatic uterine fibroids.[4] These patients can be managed expectantly with frequent clinical examinations and pelvic ultrasounds to monitor both the adnexa and the uterine size. Changes in the course of the disease warrant an investigation and will dictate treatment decisions.

Medical management

Medical management of uterine fibroids is an approach which has a great deal of appeal because of its relative ease compared to surgery. Indications for therapy are similar to surgical intervention and would center on preserving fertility potential or an individual's desire to maintain her uterus. Discussion of this option does not preclude definitive therapy, which at the present time involves surgery.

The decision to preserve a uterus may be addressed as an aspect of age, but in an era where grandmothers carry and deliver their grandchildren or a 60-year-old can deliver a child through donated oocytes, age becomes quite "relative". One must also address cultural norms in that a woman who has her uterus removed and becomes amenorrheic is considered "old" in some areas of the world.

Aspects of symptoms must be clearly addressed so that bleeding can be described and a determination of the medical necessity can be made. Other facts, such as abdominal pain, pressure, and effect on bowel and bladder function must be assessed. Irregular vaginal bleeding is by far the most common complaint (30%).[3] The examinations other than the physical examination which may be performed are ultrasound and possibly MRI. Endometrial biopsy is another tool that can help focus the explanation of the etiology of bleeding.

In women who wish conservative management, the approach will be how we can use medical therapy. If there is irregular bleeding and the endometrial biopsy is negative, cyclic hormones such as birth control pills or progestin can be tried. It seems that these hormones do not affect the growth of the myomas. In fact, myomas have been noted to decrease in size by 46%.[26] In many cases, the oral hormones may help the bleeding. Another report also supports no association between fibroid growth and oral contraceptive use with an RR of 1.1 in ever vs. never users (with 95% confidence interval (CI) of 0.8–1.5).[28] Progestin contraceptive pills or other progestin such as medroxyprogesterone or norethindrone either cyclically or continuously may be used to regulate the patient's cyclic bleeding.

Estrogen

Leiomyomata are sensitive to hyperestrogenic states such as pregnancy and the luteal phase. Compared to adjacent myometrium, myomas appear to have an increased number of estrogen receptors.[29–34] Protein levels in the myoma are threefold higher compared to myometrial tissue.[34] Animal studies support the effects of estrogen on fibroid growth.[35-38] Estrogen stimulates and tamoxifen, an anti-estrogen, inhibits the growth of these tumors.[35]

Changes in local estrogen biosynthesis may also play a role. Leiomyomas have been found to express cytochrome p19 and its product p450 aromatase mRNA at levels detected in adipose tissue. Interestingly, p450 aromatase transcripts were not found in myometrium of women without myomas; whereas, expression was found in myometrium of tissue adjacent to myomas but at levels 1.5 to 2.5-fold lower than in the tumors themselves. Leiomyomas have been shown to convert androstenedione to estrone, a less potent estrogen than estradiol.[39] There has also been some variation in different racial groups with an increased number of estrogen and progesterone receptors noted in Caucasian patients.[40]

It is clear that myoma size increases with estrogen and regresses after menopause. There are several reports of increased size on clomiphene and tamoxifen therapy. In individual cases, myomas were noted to increase with clomiphene (two of two)[41,42] and with tamoxifen (13 of 21) myomas.[43] In another study, oral tamoxifen was combined with gonadotropin-releasing hormone analog (GnRHa) (goserelin) after an initial six months agonist therapy, and there was no further reduction in size with the combined regimen for an additional six months.[44] Although an increase in myoma size is not routinely seen, women on tamoxifen therapy need close follow-up.

GnRH analogs have been used to treat leiomyoma through the down-regulation and desensitization of the hypothalamic–pituitary axis resulting in a "reversible" hypo-estrogen state.[45-60] The agonists were long acting compared to the native GnRH that had a half-life of hours.[45] Initially, it was thought that the leiomyomas would decrease in size and take a longer time to return to their original size, but this was not true for a large proportion of patients.[57,58] It has been suggested that myomas may be reduced and 17% may have no symptoms after the effect is resolved.[61]

Even though our chapter focuses on conservative management, effects and benefits of preoperative

Table 8.1. Possible benefits from GnRH analog therapy of uterine myomas[59,60]

Adjunct to Hysterectomy
- Decrease in uterine size and blood flow
- Vaginal or laparoscopy versus laparotomy
- Decrease intraoperative blood loss
- Pfannensteil versus vertical incision
- Decrease injury to adjacent organs
- Increase preoperative hematocrit
- Allow autologous blood donation
- Decrease the need for transfusion

Adjunct to Myomectomy
- Possible decrease in size and blood loss
- May facilitate endoscopic resection
- May allow pfannensteil incision .
- May decrease adjacent tissue injury
- Increase hematocrit
- Autologous donation and decrease need for transfusion

therapy are listed in Table 8.1. It suggests the benefits of preoperative therapy, particularly for anemia. Instead of laparotomy, the smaller uterine fibroids may be amenable to vaginal or laparoscopic hysterectomy. Intra-operative blood loss is decreased.[54,62] Improvement of hematocrit secondary to GnRHa treatment has been noted in anemic patients compared to iron therapy alone.[63] This allows autologous donation and reduces the risk of transfusion. If endoscopic surgery is planned, it may facilitate laparoscopic and hysteroscopic resection. The reduction in size is 40–60% of the original volume with two to six months treatment. With 2 months GnRHa, there was little change in triglycerides and lipoproteins levels.[64]

The most common side effect of GnRHa is hot flushes seen in nearly all patients. Irregular vaginal bleeding, headache, depression, insomnia and myalgias are found in ≤15% of patients. Table 8.2 depicts side effects of GnRHa.[60] GnRHa may be helpful in many cases but it is important to balance the therapy, side effects, cost, and surgical plan. In a study published in 2001, a combination of tibolone and GnRHa was compared to GnRHa alone and no benefit was noted at laparoscopic surgery.[65]

Table 8.2. Hypo-estrogenic side effects with GnRH analog use[60]

- 75–100% of cases ⟶ hot flushes
- 20–40% of cases ⟶ irregular vaginal bleeding
- 5–15% of cases ⟶ headache, insomnia, vaginal dryness, weight change, depression, myalgia/arthralgia, hair loss, edema
- 0–2% of cases ⟶ vaginal bleeding, allergic reaction

Progestins and Progesterone

Progesterone receptors have been found in increased numbers in leiomyomas compared to adjacent myometrium. In the progesterone-dominated luteal phase, myoma is larger and mitotic activity increases. These findings suggest a role of progesterone in the growth of leiomyomas. Increased progesterone receptor mRNA and protein have been noted also in myoma.[66,67] There are two forms of progesterone receptor (A and B) with a predominance of A.[68–70] Clinical studies on the effects of progestins and progesterone on leiomyomas have been conflicting.[66,71,72] One study reported more receptors in younger than in older women and there were more mitotic figures in the early secretory phase.[73] Others could not confirm it, although they showed an increase of estrogen receptors.[74,75]

The use of progesterone 20 mg/day is associated with a subjective decrease in the uterine fibroids, but not on radiologic examination. More recent studies demonstrated that treatment with three months antiprogesterone (RU-486) decreased uterine size by 52%. Amenorrhea was induced in all patients and although there were hot flushes reported in two of 10 patients, estrogen levels remained normal.[76,77] Under in vitro conditions, progestin did not appear to affect the expression of connexin 43 gene expression in leiomyoma and myometrial primary cell culture.[78]

Androgens

The relationship between myoma and androgens or androgenic agents remains unclear. One study suggested that increased concentrations of 5-alpha androgens implied androgen sensitivity of these tissues.[79] Several small studies have used Danazol and one noted no effect on the myoma,[80,81] and in the other there was a 20% reduction in size. In the latter study, androgen side effects led to discontinuation of the treatment.[81] The authors suggested that the lack of reduction in size could be due to the anabolic effects of Danazol.

Gestrinone has also been used as a preoperative adjunct, and it has anti-estrogenic and antiprogesterone effects. Studies have reported that 76–96% of women have amenorrhea and improvement in their symptoms. Various doses of gestrinone and routes of administration have been reported. The limiting factor of use has been androgenic side effects with up to 93% experiencing acne and seborrhea. Also, up to 24% of patients reported myalgia and/or arthralgia.[82–85] Reduction of uterine volume of 40% was noted after 12 months of therapy and regrowth after discontinuance was slow.[85] Further study may be necessary to more clearly establish relationships of androgens in myoma therapy.

Hypoestrogenism plus estrogen/progestin add back therapy

A different treatment strategy is the use of GnRHa to reduce the estrogen level, then adding back various estrogens or progestin to reduce the side effects. While this method may not be applicable to all patients, it is an alternative treatment for poor surgical candidates or women desiring minimal therapy until menopause. It is important to remember that even though the chance for malignancy is low, it will increase to about 0.5% in the older women.[14,86] In one study, a group received leuprolide acetate and another received a combination of leuprolide and medroxyprogesterone acetate. After six months, the group receiving medroxyprogesterone in addition had only a 14% reduction.[51] Medroxyprogesterone reduced hot flushes.[87]

Administration of leuprolide acetate for three months is associated with a 49% reduction in volume. Additional 0.625 mg conjugated estrogen daily with 10 days of 10 mg of medroxyprogesterone for another 24 months results in no change in uterine size.[53,57] One patient required 1.25 conjugated estrogen to relieve all of her symptoms. All had regular withdrawal bleeding and no loss of bone density.[54]

Another analog, goserelin, was studied in a similar manner obtaining a hypoestrogenic state in 10 women for three months, then 0.3 mg conjugated estrogen was given cyclically with 5 mg medroxyprogesterone for 10 days. The reduction in myoma size was 49%, which was maintained during the add-back regiment. However, the hypoestrogenic side effects were not well controlled.[88] The combination of GnRH analog and tamoxifen have been discussed previously. These regimens are proposed to work through an estrogen threshold hypothesis that suggests that if the threshold is not exceeded, benefits from both ends of the spectrum can be maintained.[89]

The future of medical treatment

In contrast to GnRHa, GnRH antagonists have no initial stimulatory effect and are a promising treatment for uterine myoma. The use of calcium or bisphosphonates to minimize bone loss in patients treated with GnRHa or antagonist may be helpful. The manipulation of growth factors, vaccines and genetics may well develop a role in the treatment of these common uterine tumors. It is important to address the specific issues of therapy as they relate to the individual patient and her desired outcome.

REFERENCES

1. Cramer S & Patel A (1990). The frequency of uterine leiomyomas. *Am J Clin Pathol* **94**: 435–8.
2. Farquhar C & Steiner C (2002). Hysterectomy rates in the United States 1990–1997. *Obstet Gynecol* **99**: 229–34.
3. Carlson K, Miller B & Fowler F (1994). The Maine women's health study: II. Outcomes of non-surgical management of leiomyomas, abnormal bleeding and chronic pelvic pain. *Obstet Gynecol* **83**: 566–72.
4. *Management of Uterine Fibroids. Summary, Evidence Report/Technology Assessment.* January 2001, *Healthcare Assessment* No. 34 (AHRQ Publication No. 01-E051). Rockville, MD: Agency for Healthcare Research and Quality.
5. Van Voohis J, DeWaay D, Syrop C, et al. (2002). Natural history of uterine polyps and fibroids. *J Soc Gynecol Invest* **9**: 348A.
6. Vardi J & Tovell H (1980). Leiomyosarcoma of the uterus: Clinicopathologic study. *Obstet Gynecol* **56**: 428–34.
7. Parker W, Fu Y, Berek J (1994). Uterine sarcoma in patients operated on for presumed leiomyoma and rapidly growing leiomyoma. *Obstet Gynecol* **83**: 414–18.
8. Varol N, Healey M, Tang P, et al. (2001). Ten-year review of hysterectomy morbidity and mortality: Can we change direction? *Aust NZ J Obstet Gynecol* **41**: 295–302.
9. Virtanen H & Makinen J (1995). Mortality after gynecologic operations in Finland. *Br J Obstet Gynecol* **102**: 54–7.
10. Kahanpaa K, Wahlstrom T, Grohn P, et al. (1986). Sarcomas of the uterus: a clinicopathologic study of 119 patients. *Obstet Gynecol* **67**: 417–24.
11. Barbieri R (1999). Ambulatory management of uterine leiomyomata. *Clin Obstet Gynecol* **42**: 196–205.
12. Kawamura N, Ichimura T, Ito F, et al. (2002). Transcervical needle biopsy for the differential diagnosis between uterine sarcoma and leiomyoma. *Cancer* **94**: 1713–20.
13. Mesia A, Williams F, Yan Z, et al. (1998). Aborted leiomyosarcoma after treatment with leuprolide acetate. *Obstet Gynecol* **92**: 664–6.
14. Liebsohn S, d'Ablaing G, Mishell D, et al. (1990). Leiomyosarcoma in a series of hysterectomies performed for presumed uterine leiomyomas. *Am J Obstet Gynecol* **162**: 968–76.
15. *Ovarian cancer: screening, treatment and follow-up: NIH consensus statement,* (1994) April 5–7; **12**(3): 30.
16. Richardson G, Scully R & Nikrui N (1985). Common epithelial cancer of the ovary. *New Eng J Med* **312**: 415–19.
17. Reiter R, Wagner P & Gambrose I (1992). Routine hysterectomy for large asymptomatic uterine leiomyomata: a reappraisal. *Obstet Gynecol* **79**: 481–4.
18. Hillis S, Marchbanks P & Peterson H (1996). Uterine size and risk of complications among women undergoing abdominal hysterectomy for leiomyomas. *Obstet Gynecol* **87**: 539–43.
19. Stewart E, Faur A, Wise L, et al. (2002). Predictors of subsequent surgery for uterine leiomyomata after abdominal myomectomy. *Obstet Gynecol* **99**: 426–32.
20. Buttram V & Reiter R (1981). Uterine leiomyomata – etiology, symptomatology and management. *Fertil Steril* **36**: 433–45.
21. Li T, Mortimer R, Cooke I (1999). Myomectomy: A retrospective study to examine reproductive performance before and after surgery. *Hum Reprod* **14**: 1735–40.
22. Bajekal N, Li T (2000). Fibroids, infertility and pregnancy wastage. *Hum Reprod Update* **6**: 614–20.
23. Verkauf B (1992). Myomectomy for fertility enhancement and preservation. *Fertil Steril* **58**: 1–15.
24. Vergani P, Ghidini A, Strobelt N, et al. (1994). Do uterine

leiomyomas influence pregnancy outcome? *Am J Perinatol* **11**: 356–8.

25. Coronado G, Marshall L & Schwarz S (2000). Complications in pregnancy, labor and delivery with uterine leiomyomas: a population-based study. *Obstet Gynecol* **95**: 764–9.

26. Ang W, Farrell E, Vollenhoven B, et al. (2001). Effect of hormone replacement therapies and selective receptor modulators in postmenopausal women with uterine leiomyomas: A literature review. *Climateric* **4**: 284–92.

27. Palomba S, Sena T, Noia R, et al. (2001). Transdermal hormone replacement therapy in postmenopausal women with uterine leiomyomas. *Obstet Gynecol* **98**: 1053–8.

28. Parazzini R, Negri E, La Vecchia C, et al. (1992). Oral contraceptive use and risk of uterine fibroids. *Obstet Gynecol* **79**: 430–3.

29. Tamaya T, Fujimoto J, Okada H, et al. (1985) Composition of cellular levels of steroid receptors in uterine leiomyomata and myometrium. *Acta Obstet Gynecol Scand* **64**: 307–9.

30. Nardelli G, Mega M, Bertasi M, et al. (1987). Estradiol and progesterone binding in uterine leiomyomata and pregnant myometrium. *Clin Exp Obstet Gynecol* **14**: 155–60.

31. Chrapusta S, Konopka B, et al. (1990). Immunoreactive and estrogen-binding estrogen receptors and progestin receptor levels in uterine leiomyomata and their parental myometrium. *Eur J Gynecol Oncol* **11**: 275–81.

32. Chrapusta S, Sienski W, Konopka B, et al. (1990). Estrogen and progesterone receptor levels in uterine leiomyomata: relation to the tumor histology and the phase of the menstrual cycle. *Eur J Gynecol Oncol* **11**: 381–7.

33. Han K, Lee W, Harris C, et al. (1994). Comparison of chromosome aberrations in leiomyoma and leiomyosarcoma using FISH on archival tissues. *Cancer Genet Cyto Genet* **74**: 19–24.

34. Brandon D, Erickson T, Keenan E, et al. (1995) Estrogen receptor gene expression in human uterine leiomyomata. *Clin Endocrinol* **80**: 1876–81.

35. Howe S, Gottardis M, Everitt J, et al. (1995). Rodent model of reproductive tract leiomyomata. Establishment and characterization of tumor-derived cell lines. *Am J Path* **146**: 1568–79.

36. Howe S, Gottardis M, Everitt J, et al. (1994). Estrogen stimulation and tamoxifen inhibition of leiomyomata cell growth in vitro and in vivo. *Endocrinol* **136**: 4996–5003.

37. Gibson J, Sells D, Cheng H, et al. (1987). Induction of uterine leiomyomas in mice by medrozalol and prevention by propranolol. *Toxicol Pathol* **4**: 468–73.

38. Porter K, Tsibris J, Nicosia S, et al. (1995). Estrogen-induced guinea pig model for uterine leiomyomas: Do the ovaries protect? *Bio Reprod* **52**: 824–32.

39. Bulum S, Simpson E, Word R, et al. (1994). Expression of the CY 19 gene and its products aromatase cytochrome P450 in human uterine leiomyoma tissue and cells in culture. *J Clinc Endo Metab* **78**: 736–43.

40. Sadon O, Iddekinge B, Savage N, et al. (1988). Ethnic variation in estrogen and progesterone receptor concentrations in leiomyoma and normal myometrium. *Gynecol Endocrinol* **2**: 275–82.

41. Frankel T & Benjamin F (1973). Rapid enlargement of uterine fibroid after clomiphene therapy. *J Obstet Gynecol BR Commonwealth* **80**: 764.

42. Felmingham J & Corcoran R (1975). Rapid enlargement of uterine fibroid after clomiphene therapy (letter). *Br J Obstet Gynecol* **82**: 431–2.

43. Schwartz L, Rutkowski N, Horan C, et al. (1998). Use of transvaginal ultrasonography to monitor the effects of tamoxifen on uterine leiomyoma size and ovarian cyst formation. *J Ultrasound Med* **17**: 699–703.

44. Lumsden M, West C, Hillier H, et al. (1989). Estrogenic action of tamoxifen in women treated with LHRH (goserelin) lack of shrinkage in uterine fibroids. *Fertil Steril* **52**: 924–9.

45. Filicori M, Hall D, Loughlin J, et al. (1983). A conservative approach to the management of uterine leiomyomata: pituitary desensitization by a utilizing hormone-releasing hormone analogue. *Am J Obstet Gynecol* **147**: 726–7.

46. Healy D, Lawson S, Abbott M, et al. (1986). Toward removing uterine fibroids without surgery: subcutaneous infusion of a luteinizing hormone-releasing hormone agonist commencing in the luteal phase. *J Clinc Endo Metab* **63**: 619–25.

47. Maheux R, Guilloteau C, Lemay A, et al. (1985). Luteinizing hormone-releasing hormone agonist and uterine leiomyoma: a pilot study. *Am J Obstet Gynecol* **152**: 1034–8.

48. Van Leusden H. (1986). Rapid reduction of uterine myomas after short term treatment with microencapsulated D-Trp6-LHRH. *Lancet* **2**: 1213.

49. Coddington C, Collins R, Shawker T, et al. (1986). Long acting gonadotropin hormone-releasing hormone analog used to treat uteri. *Fertil Steril* **45**: 624–9.

50. West C, Lumsden M, Lawson S, et al. (1987). Shrinkage of uterine fibroids during therapy with goserelin: a luteinizing hormone-releasing hormone agonist administered as a monthly subcutaneous depot. *Fertil Steril* **48**: 45–51.

51. Friedman A, Barbieri R, Doubilet P, et al. (1988). A randomized double blind trial of gonadotropin-releasing hormone agonist (leuprolide) with or without medroxyprogesterone acetate in treatment of leiomyomata uteri. *Fertil Steril* **49**: 404.

52. Lumsden M, West C & Baird D (1987). Goserelin therapy before surgery for uterine fibroids. *Lancet* **1**: 36–7.

53. Friedman A, Harrison-Atlas D, Barbieri R, et al. (1989).

A randomized placebo controlled double blinded study evaluating the efficacy of leuprolide acetate depot in the treatment of uterine leiomyomata. *Fertil Steril* **51**: 251.

54. Friedman A, Rein M & Harrison-Atlas D (1989). A randomized placebo controlled double blind study evaluating leuprolide acetate depot treatment before myomectomy. *Fertil Steril* **52**: 728–33.

55. Andreyko J, Blumfield Z, Marshall L, et al. (1988). Use of an agonist analog of gonadotropin-releasing hormone (hefarelin) to treat leiomyomas: assessment by magnetic resonance imaging. *Am J Obstet Gynecol* **158**: 903–10.

56. Matta W, Shaw R & Nye M. (1989) Long term follow-up of patients with uterine fibroids after treatment with the LHRH agonist buserelin. *Br J Obstet Gynecol* **96**: 200–6.

57. Friedman A, Hoffman D, Comite F, et al. (1991). Treatment of uterine leiomyomata with leuprolide acetate depot: a double blind placebo controlled multimember study. *Obstet Gynecol* **77**: 720–5.

58. Letterie G, Coddingington C, Winkel C, et al. (1989). Efficacy of gonadotropin-releasing hormone agonist in the treatment of uterine leiomyomata: long term follow-up. *Fertil Steril* **51**: 951–6.

59. Stewart E & Friedman A (1992). Steroidal treatment of myomas: Preoperative and long term medical therapy. *Sem Reprod Endo* **10**: 344–57.

60. Barbieri R & Friedman A (1991). *Gonadotropin Releasing Hormone Analogs: Applications in Gynecology.* New York: Elsevier Science Publishing.

61. Fedele L, Vercellini P, Bianchi S, et al. (1990). Treatment with GnRH agonists before myomectomy and the risk of short term myoma recurrence. *Br J Obstet Gynecol* **97**: 393–6.

62. Stovall T, Ling F, Henry L, et al. (1991) A randomized trial evaluating leuprolide acetate before hysterectomy as treatment for leiomyomas. *Am J Obstet Gynecol* **164**: 1420–3.

63. Stovall T (1995). GnRH agonist and iron versus placebo and iron in the anemic patient before surgery for leiomyomas: a randomized controlled trial. Leuprolide acetate study group. *Obstet Gynecol* **86**: 65–71.

64. Coddington C, Brzyski R, Hansen K, et al. (1992). Short term treatment with leuprolide acetate is a successful adjunct to surgical therapy of leiomyomata uteri. *Surg Gynecol Obstet* **175**: 57.

65. Palomba S, Pellicano M, Affinito P, et al. (2001). Effectiveness of short-term administration of tibolone plus gonadotropin releasing hormone analogue on the surgical outcome of laparoscopic myomectomy. *Fertil Steril* **75**: 429–33.

66. Rein M, Barbieri R & Friedman A (1995). Progesterone: a critical role in the pathogenesis of uterine myomas. *Am J Obstet Gynecol* **172**: 14–18.

67. Brandon D, Bethers C, Strawn E, et al. (1993). Progesterone receptor messenger ribonucleic acid and protein are over expressed in human uterine leiomyomas. *Am J Obstet Gynecol* **169**: 78–85.

68. Stewart E, Austin D, Jain P, et al. (1996). RU486 suppresses prolactin production in explant cultures of leiomyoma and myometrium. *Fertil Steril* **65**: 1119–24.

69. Fujimoto J, Ichigo S, Hori M, et al. (1995). Expression of progesterone receptor A and B mRNAs in gynecologic tumors. *Tumor Biol* **16**: 254–60.

70. Vegeto E, Shahbaz M, Wen D, et al. (1993). Human progesterone receptor A form is a cell-and-promoter-specific repressor of progesterone receptor B function. *Mol Endocrinol* **7**: 1244–55.

71. Carr B, Marshburn P, Weatherall P, et al. (1993). An evaluation of the effect of gonadotropin releasing hormone analogs and medroxyprogesterone acetate on uterine leiomyoma volume by MRI: A prospective, randomized, double blind, placebo controlled cross over trial. *J Clinc Endo Metab* **76**: 1217–33.

72. Harrison-Woolrych M & Robinson R (1995). Fibroid growth in response to high-dose progestogen. *Fertil Steril* **64**: 191–7.

73. Kawaguchi K (1989). Mitotic activity in uterine leiomyomas during the menstrual cycle. *Am J Obstet Gynecol* **160**: 637–41.

74. Wilson E & Yang F (1980). Estradiol and progesterone binding in uterine leiomyoma and in normal uterine tissues. *Obstet Gynecol* **55**: 20–4.

75. Soules M & McCarty K (1982). Leiomyomas: Steroid receptor content. Variations within the normal menstrual cycles. *Am J Obstet Gynecol* **143**: 6–11.

76. Murphy A, Kettel M, Morales A, et al. (1993). Regression of uterine myomata to anti-progesterone RU486. *J Clinc Endo Metab* **76**: 513.

77. Murphy A, Morales A, Kettel M, et al. (1995). Regression of uterine leiomyomata to anti-progesterone RU486: dose response effect. *Fertil Steril* **64**: 187.

78. Zhao K, Kupperman L & Geimonen E (1996). Progestin represses human connexin 43 gene expression similar in primary cultures of myometrial and leiomyomas. *Bio Reprod* **54**: 607–15.

79. Reddy V & Rose L (1979). Delta 4-3-ketosteroid 5-alpha-oxidoreductase in human uterine leiomyoma. *Am J Obstet Gynecol* **1979**: 415–18.

80. DeCherney A, Maheux R & Polan M (1983). A medical treatment for myomata uteri. *Fertil Steril* **39**: 429–30.

81. Yuen B (1981). Danazol and uterine leiomyomas. *Can J Med Assoc* **124**: 963–4.

82. Coutinho E (1989). Gestrinone in the treatment of myomas. *Acta Obstet Gynecol Scand* **150**(Suppl.): 39–46.

83. Coutinho E (1990). Treatment of large fibroids with high doses of gestrinone. *Gynecol Obstet Invest* **30**: 44–7.

84. Coutinho E, Boulanger G & Goncalves M (1986). Regression of uterine leiomyomas after treatment with gestrinone, and anti-estrogen, anti-progesterone. *Am J Obstet Gynecol* **155**: 761–7.

85. Coutinho E & Concalves M (1989). Long term treatment of leiomyomas with gestrinone. *Fertil Steril* **51**: 939–46.

86. Montague A, Swartz D & Woodruff D (1965). Sarcoma arising in leiomyoma of uterus: Factors affecting prognosis. *Am J Obstet Gynecol* **92**: 421.

87. Schiff L, Tulchinsky D, Cramer D, et al. (1990). Oral medroxyprogesterone in the treatment of post-menopausal symptoms. *JAMA* **224**: 1443–5.

88. Maheux R, Lemay A, Blanchet P, et al. (1991). Maintained reduction of uterine leiomyoma following addition of hormonal replacement therapy to a monthly luteinizing hormone releasing agonist implant: a pilot study. *Hum Reprod* **6**: 500–5.

89. Friedman A, Lobel S, Rein M, et al. (1990). Efficacy and safety considerations in women with uterine leiomyomas treated with gonadtropin-releasing hormone agonists: The estrogen threshold hypothesis. *Am J Obstet Gynecol* **163**: 1114–19.

9

Hysterectomy for uterine fibroid

Haya Al-Fozan and Togas Tulandi

McGill University, Montreal, Quebec, Canada

The most common indication for hysterectomy is uterine fibroids. It is estimated that approximately one-third of all hysterectomies are done for problems related to uterine fibroids.[1,2] The clinical indications vary from merely the presence of fibroid to menorrhagia, pressure symptoms, infertility, or habitual abortion.

In many instances they are asymptomatic, but in some women they may be associated with heavy menstrual bleeding, infertility, pressure symptoms, and miscarriage. Hysterectomy can be performed abdominally, laparoscopically, or vaginally, and could be total or subtotal. The approach of the procedure is determined by the clinical situation, the preference and the expertise of the surgeon, and to a certain extent by the patient's desire. In this review we will discuss the risks and benefits of different types of hysterectomy in the treatment of uterine fibroid.

Abdominal hysterectomy

Total abdominal hysterectomy (TAH) remains the conventional treatment for uterine fibroids in women who have completed their family. In the United States, 75% of all hysterectomies are done by laparotomy,[3] which is threefold higher than that for vaginal hysterectomy (VH).[2] TAH is a major operation with three to five days of hospitalization and a convalescence time of several weeks. It is associated with major morbidity in 3% and minor morbidity in about 14% of cases.[4] However, it is a well-received operation with as many as 85–90% of women being satisfied with the procedure and reporting improved quality of life.[5]

Compared to that of VH (27%), the complication rate of abdominal hysterectomy is 49%.[2] It depends on several factors. For example, uterine size of > 500 g is associated with an increased risk of TAH with a twofold increase in the probability of hemorrhage requiring transfusion.[6] In order to reduce the size of the uterus and the fibroids, preoperative treatment with gonadotropin-releasing hormone analog (GnRHas) has been advocated. A smaller uterus allows conduct of hysterectomy by vaginal or laparoscopic approach. Other advantages of GnRHa are improved hematological status due to the absence of vaginal bleeding during the treatment, and decreased blood loss during surgery.[6]

Vaginal hysterectomy

The rate of VH in women with uterine fibroid has been reported to be as low as 4%.[1] The abdominal approach for hysterectomy for myomas has been traditionally preferred because the vaginal approach is technically more difficult. However, compared to TAH, vaginal hysterectomy is associated with lower complication rates, shorter hospital stay and convalescence, lower in-patient hospital cost, and better quality of life outcomes.[2,7–9]

However, a large uterine fibroid has to be first morcellated and this can be difficult and may result in complications. Accordingly, vaginal hysterectomy should be performed on selected cases of uterine fibroids. In properly selected patients with some degree of uterine descent, blood loss and the operative morbidity related to VH are equal to that of TAH.

The vaginal surgeon should be familiar with morcellation, and should be able to convert to TAH if needed.[10] Mazdisnian et al.[11] found that myoma location was more important than absolute uterine size. In their series, five of seven patients with unsuccessful VH had large lower segment myomas preventing uterine descent. It seems that the failure rate is related to the presence of large cervical myoma.[12]

Factors affecting the choice of VH

Uterine size

The upper limit of uterine size for VH depends on the surgeon's experience and preference. In general, VH can be done for a uterus of <12 weeks gestational size (280 g). On the other hand, Kovac[13] reported that uteri much larger than the 280 g could be removed vaginally if the surgeon has the expertise in the techniques of morcellation, bivalving and coring. Darai et al.[14] found that they had no difficulties with VH if the uterine weight was <500 g.

Concomitant pathology

Patients with a history or clinical findings suggestive of endometriosis, adnexal disease, chronic pelvic pain, adhesions, previous pelvic surgery or chronic pelvic inflammatory disease are better candidates for laparoscopic hysterectomy than VH.[15] It is indeed difficult, if not impossible, to assess the pathology of these concomitants by the vaginal approach. Some authors, however, reported that they have performed VH in these types of patients uneventfully.[16,17]

Age

Patients of ≥50 years of age have more chance of a successful outcome if they undergo VH, as uterine prolapse is more common in this age group.[18]

Laparoscopic hysterectomy

Laparoscopic assisted vaginal hysterectomy (LAVH)

LAVH has emerged as a viable surgical option to abdominal hysterectomy. Nevertheless, there are no advantages of LAVH over the vaginal approach when there is no contraindication to VH. In fact, LAVH is associated with a longer operating time.[7,12] Compared to laparotomy, LAVH offers the benefits of laparoscopic surgery including smaller incision, shorter hospitalization, less pain, and rapid recovery.[19]

In theory, LAVH can replace many abdominal hysterectomies for large fibroid uteri when VH is not feasible.[20] The laparoscopic approach allows liberation of adhesions, excision of endometriosis, and a thorough evaluation of the abdominal cavity.[21,22] It is helpful when the vaginal access is severely reduced or the mobility of the uterus is limited. Yen et al.[23] found that coagulation of the uterine vessels and supracervical amputation of the uterus by laparoscopy followed by trachelectomy are helpful to reduce the operating time and the blood loss. The mean uterine weight in their study was 517.3 g.

Laparoscopic hysterectomy (LH)

LH is a substitute for TAH, but not for VH[23] (Figure 9.1). It is associated with a longer operating time, but in the hands of expert laparoscopic surgeons, most LHs can be done within two hours. The upper limit of uterine size depends on the surgeon's experience and preference (Figure 9.2, see also color plates). In dealing with a large uterus, the trocars should placed higher than the uterine fundus. Our upper limit of uterine size is 18 gestational weeks. The uterus can be reduced in size by enucleation or morcellation of the myomas, coring of the central part of the uterus, or by bisection.[24] In our experience, lateral enlargement of the uterus plays a more important role than that of the uterine size. Access to the uterine vessels is very difficult or impossible in the presence of marked enlargement of the uterus laterally.

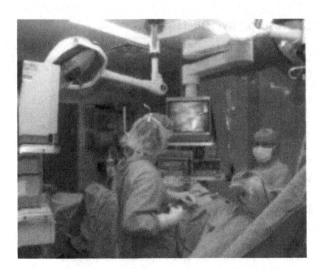

Figure 9.1. Operating room set-up for laparoscopic hysterectomy.

Total versus subtotal hysterectomy

In the past decade, subtotal or supracervical hysterectomy has regained popularity. This is due to several reasons including less injury to the ureter and less disruption of autonomic nervous pathways. Furthermore, it is now possible to detect cervical abnormalities in the early stages.

Supracervical hysterectomy is associated with less wound infections, hematomas, and urinary tract infection. Vault granulation that occurred in about 21% of total hysterectomies will not be found after subtotal hysterectomy.[25] Subtotal hysterectomy is particularly suitable for removal of fibroid uterus providing that the cervical pathology is always normal. On the other hand, women with cervical myoma are better candidates for total hysterectomy. Milad et al.[26] found that compared to LAVH, laparoscopic supracervical hysterectomy is associated with shorter operating times, and a shorter hospital stay.

Bladder function

Both sympathetic and parasympathetic innervations reach the bladder via the pelvic plexus through the cardinal ligament and the Frankenhauser's plexus. These innervations are potentially susceptible to damage during paracervical dissection in total hysterectomy.[27] Also women who had had total hysterectomy experienced more urinary frequency than those who had undergone supracervical hysterectomy.[28] Others could not confirm these findings.[29] To date, there is insufficient information about bladder function after supracervical hysterectomy than there is for total hysterectomy.[27]

Sexual function

Disturbance of the innervations of the cervix and the upper vagina after total hysterectomy could interfere with lubrication and orgasm.[25] Kilkku et al.[30] noted that the frequency of orgasm was significantly reduced one year after surgery in the total hysterectomy group while it remained unchanged in the subtotal group. Others suggested that the magnitude of a negative effect of total hysterectomy on sexual function is not as great as originally perceived.[29]

Sexual function depends on several factors, including cultural beliefs and education, and it is difficult to relate it mainly to the type of hysterectomy.

Risk of cervical cancer

Prevention of cervical carcinoma is a benefit for women undergoing total hysterectomy. However, although removal of the cervix reduces the risk of cervical cancer, there is still a small risk of preinvasive and invasive neoplasia of the vaginal vault. The incidence of cervical stump carcinoma was 0.4% before the initiation of cervical screening (Papanicolaou test) and 0.1% thereafter.[31] The risk of cervical carcinoma following a supracervical hysterectomy and electrocoagulation of the endocervical canal was also about 0.1%.[32] This is similar to the incidence of vaginal vault malignancy after a total hysterectomy.[31]

Outcomes

Abdominal and vaginal hysterectomy

In general, postoperative morbidity of vaginal hysterectomy is more favorable than TAH.[2,9] It is associated with mortality similar to TAH, but is

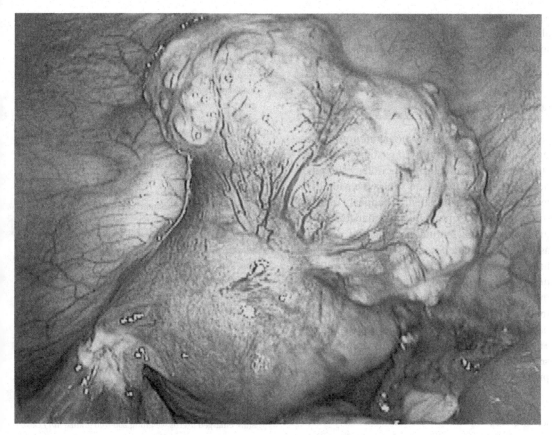

Figure 9.2. Uterus before laparoscopic hysterectomy. A calcified subserous myoma is shown. The patient also had a large cervical myoma (not seen). See also color plates.

associated with less morbidity, shorter hospital stay and lower cost.[10] Yet, in women with uterine myomas, the abdominal approach has been more popular because the vaginal approach is technically more difficult and riskier. VH results in better quality of life outcome and lower utilization and cost compared to abdominal hysterectomy.[8,33]

Laparoscopic assisted vaginal hysterectomy (LAVH)

The main role of LAVH is not to replace simple vaginal hysterectomy, but to decrease the frequency of TAH. The outcome of LAVH is superior to that of TAH with respect to complication rate, postoperative pain, duration of hospitalization, and the return to normal activity.[34,35] However, it is associated with a longer operating time.[7,12] Although some authors have reported a higher cost for LAVH, Falcone et al.[36] found that the hospital costs of LAVH are similar to that of TAH. Abenhaim et al.[8] found that compared to the abdominal and the vaginal approach, the laparoscopic hysterectomy is associated with higher operating room costs but the hospital stay is shorter and the nursing fee is lower. This results in lower total in-hospital costs.

Laparoscopic hysterectomy

Improvement of laparoscopic techniques has made it possible to remove the uterus entirely by laparoscopy. In a large analysis of over 160 000 hysterectomies among 180 hospitals, the total complication rates of abdominal, vaginal, and laparoscopic hysterectomy were 9.1%, 7.8%, and 8.8% respectively.[37]

Conclusions

For diseases above the cervix such as uterine fibroids, subtotal or supracervical hysterectomy is particularly suitable. However, cervical cytology should be normal for at least three years. Otherwise, a total hysterectomy can be considered. VH appears to be associated with lower morbidity rates than for abdominal hysterectomy, but uterine weight of >500 g is associated with complications. With improvement in the laparoscopy techniques, the use of GnRHa to decrease the uterine and fibroid size, and the ease of uterine removal with morcellation, more hysterectomies can be performed by laparoscopy giving the patients the advantages of minimal invasive surgery. The ultimate results depend on the proper patient selection, and surgeon's experience, expertise, and preference.

REFERENCES

1. Vessey MP, Villard-Mackintosh Ll, McPherson K, et al. (1992). The epidemiology of hysterectomy. Findings in a large cohort study. *Br J Obstet Gynecol* **99**: 402–7.
2. Dicker R, Greenspan J & Strauss LT (1982). Complication of abdominal and vaginal hysterectomy among women of reproductive age in the United States. *Am J Obstet Gynecol* **144**: 841–7.
3. Wilcox LS, Koonin LM, Pokras R, et al. (1999). Hysterectomy in the United State, 1988–1990. *Obstet Gynecol* **83**: 549–55.
4. Lumsden MA, Twaddle S, Hawthorn A, et al. (2000). A randomized comparison and economic evaluation of laparoscopic assisted hysterectomy and abdominal hysterectomy. *Br J Obstet Gynecol* **107**: 1386–91.
5. Lumsden MA (2002). Embolization versus myomectomy versus hysterectomy: which is best and when? *Hum Reprod* **17**: 253–9.
6. Hillis SD, Marchbanks PA & Peterson HB (1996). Uterine size and risk of complications among women undergoing abdominal hysterectomy for leiomyomas. *Obstet Gynecol* **87**: 539–43.
7. Kovac RS (2002). Hysterectomy outcomes in patients with similar indications. *Obstet Gynecol* **95**: 787–93.
8. Abenhaim HA, Dube D, Dufort J & Tulandi T (2001). Cost analysis of laparoscopic hysterectomy, abdominal hysterectomy, and vaginal hysterectomy in Canadian teaching hospital. *JSOGC* **23**: 673–76.
9. Bachmann G (1990). Hysterectomy: a critical review. *J Reprod Med* **35**: 839–62.
10. Adamson GD (1996). Myoma, laparoscopic hysterectomy. *Infertil Reprod Med Clinics N Am* **7**: 179–207.
11. Mazdisnian F, Kurzel R, Coe S, et al. (1995). Vaginal hysterectomy by uterine morcellation: an efficient, non-morbid procedure. *Obstet Gynecol* **86**: 60.
12. Ottoson C, Ligman G & Ottoson L (2000). Three methods for hysterectomies: a randomized, prospective study of short-term outcome. *Br J Obstet Gynecol* **107**: 1380–5.
13. Kovac RS (1995). Guidelines to determine the route of hysterectomy. *Obstet Gynecol* **85**: 18.
14. Darai E, Soriano D, Kimata P, et al. (2001). Vaginal hysterectomy for enlarged uteri, with or without laparoscopic assistance: randomized study. *Obstet Gynecol* **97**: 712–16.
15. Kovac RS (1997). Which route for hysterectomy? Evidence-based outcomes guide selection. *Postgrad Med* **102**: 1–6.
16. Richardson RE, Bournas N & Magos AL (1995). Is laparoscopic hysterectomy a waste of time? *Lancet* **345**: 36–41.
17. Unger JB (1999). Vaginal hysterectomy for women with moderate enlarged uterus weighing 200–700 grams. *Am J Obstet Gynecol* **180**: 1337–44.
18. Shao JB & Wong F (2001). Factors influencing the choice of hysterectomy. *Aust NZ J Obstet Gynecol* **41**: 303–6.
19. Garry R (1997). Comparison of hysterectomy techniques and cost-benefit analysis. *Bailliere's Clinical Obstet Gynecol* **11**: 137–48.
20. Salmanli N & Maher P (1999). Laparoscopic-assisted vaginal hysterectomy for fibroid uteri weighing at least 500 grams. *Aust NZ J Obstet Gynecol* **39**: 182–4.
21. Donnez J & Nisolle M (1993). Laparoscopic supracervical (subtotal) hysterectomy (LASH). *J Gynecol Surg* **9**: 91–4.
22. Kovac SR, Cruikshank SH & Retto HF (1990). Laparoscopy assisted vaginal hysterectomy. *J Gynecol Surg* **6**: 185–93.
23. Yen Y, Liu W, Yuan C & Ng H (2002). Comparison of two procedures for laparoscopic-assisted vaginal hysterectomy of large myomatous uteri. *J Am Assoc Gynecol Laparos* **9**: 63–9.
24. Wood C & Maher PJ (1997). Laparoscopic hysterectomy. *Bailliere's Clin Obstet Gynecol* **11**: 111–36.
25. RCOG Review (1997). Bladder, bowel and sexual function

after hysterectomy for benign conditions. *Br J Obstet Gynecol* **104**: 983–7.

26. Milad MP, Morrison K, Sokl A, et al. (2001). A comparison of laparoscopic supracervical hysterectomy vs. laparoscopically assisted vaginal hysterectomy. *Surg Endos* **15**: 286–8.

27. Munro MG (1997). Supracervical hysterectomy. A time for reappraisal (clinical commentary). *Obstet Gynecol* **89**: 133–8.

28. Kilkku P (1985). Supracervical uterine amputation vs. hysterectomy with reference to subjective bladder symptoms and incontinence. *Acta Obstet Gynecol Scand* **64**: 375–9.

29. Virtanen HS, Makinen JI, Tenho T, et al. (1993). Effects of abdominal hysterectomy on urinary and sexual symptoms. *Br J Urol* **72**: 868–72.

30. Kilkku P, Gronroos M, Hirvonen T & Rauramo L (1983). Supravaginal uterine amputation vs. hysterectomy effect on libido and orgasm. *Acta Obstet Gynecol Scand* **62**: 147–52.

31. Johns A (1997). Supracervical versus total hysterectomy. *Clin Obstet Gynecol* **40**: 903–13.

32. Kilkku P & Gronroos M (1982). Preoperative electrocoagulation of the endocervical mucosal and later carcinoma of the cervical stump. *Acta Obstet Gynecol Scand* **61**: 265–8.

33. Van Den Eeden SK, Glasser M, Mathias SD, et al. (1998). Quality of life, health care utilization, and cost among women undergoing hysterectomy in a managed-care setting. *Am J Obstet Gynecol* **178**: 91–100.

34. Carter JE, Ryoo J & Katz A (1994). Laparoscopic assisted vaginal hysterectomy: a case control comparative study with total abdominal hysterectomy. *J Am Assoc Gynecol Laparos* **1**: 166.

35. Hidlebaugh D, O'Mara P & Conboy E (1994). Clinical and financial analyses of laparoscopically assisted vaginal hysterectomy versus abdominal hysterectomy. *J Am Assoc Gynecol Laparos* **1**: 357–61.

36. Falcone T, Paraiso MF & Mascha E (1999). Prospective randomized clinical trial of laparoscopically assisted vaginal hysterectomy versus total abdominal hysterectomy. *Am J Obstet Gynecol* **180**: 955–62.

37. Nezhat F, Nezhat C, Gordon S & Wilkins E (1992). Laparoscopic vs. abdominal hysterectomy. *J Reprod Med* **37**: 247–50.

10

History of embolization of uterine myoma

Jacques H. Ravina

Hopital Lariboisiere, Paris Cedex, France

In 1995, Ravina et al.[1] first reported in the English literature embolization of uterine myoma in their first 16 patients. This was a novel and unexpected therapeutic approach. The treatment options at that time were medical treatment with gonadotropin-releasing hormone analog (GnRHa), which was limited by its side effects, and surgical treatment either by myomectomy or hysterectomy. They proposed "a real alternative to surgery" namely uterine artery embolization (UAE).

Today, the value and efficacy of this treatment have been confirmed and it is widely used throughout the world. Here, I will review the process of reflection and development of UAE where gynecologists and radiologists have developed a fruitful and innovative collaboration leading to the development of UAE.

The road to innovation and development of uterine artery embolization

Arterial embolization is an interventional vascular radiology procedure that traditionally has been done for the treatment of vascular anomalies or vascular diseases of the central nervous system. Since the 1970s, it has been used also for the treatment of gastrointestinal and urinary tract bleeding.

For many years, J.J. Merland in collaboration with R. Djindjian studied and developed arterial embolization of the central nervous system at Pitie-Salpetire Hospital Paris, France. He realized that this technology could be beneficial also for other specialties. The interest of physicians in the Lariboisiere Maternity unit facilitated his intention. The first collaborative work was for the treatment of postpartum hemorrhage leading to the first publication by Pais et al. (1980).[2] However, from 1988 to 1990, few obstetricians used embolization as the treatment of postpartum bleeding. This was due to the unpredictability of the condition and the unavailability of the embolization team. Merland created a team of radiologists who were available to do embolization at short notice and this has facilitated the practical aspect of this treatment.

As a result, Lariboisiere Hospital became the Parisian center for these obstetrical emergencies. Today, embolization is accepted as one of the most effective treatments of postpartum hemorrhage. Until 1990, our hospital was the only institution in France that regularly performed hemostatic embolization. This was the basis of UAE for uterine myoma.

We began to embolize uterine myoma at about this time. Initially, we did it only to stop uterine bleeding in women with high surgical risk, such as those with extreme obesity, hypertension, vascular accidents, thromboembolism, and HIV infection. From 1990 to 1992, we treated seven women. There were three failures, in two of these women one of the uterine arteries could not be catheterized, and in the other early revascularization occurred despite two embolizations. The bleeding was controlled in three women, unfortunately they were lost from follow-up. Our intention then was to temporarily control the bleeding and reduce their disabling symptoms. We did not hope to cure these patients. The seventh patient subsequently conceived, but aborted and several months later she died due to her HIV infection.

In collaboration with J.M. Bouret and D. Fried, we studied the blood supply to the myoma by injecting dye into the uterine arteries and found that myoma almost always received a blood supply from both uterine arteries. The results of our study confirmed the forgotten and yet remarkable work by Sampson in 1912.[3] We presented our study at the meeting of the International Federation of Gynecology and Obstetrics in Montreal, and also in Dublin where we received the first prize award. Gynecologists began to rediscover the blood supply of myomata.

Our main goal then was to avoid hysterectomy in young and childless women with large uterine myomata. We aimed to embolize the uterine arteries in order to perform conservative surgical treatment of the myoma with less blood loss. We conducted the study in Bichat and Lariboisiere hospitals. We were impressed by the excellent hemostasis and none of the patients required blood transfusion. The postoperative recovery was uneventful in all patients.

Our publication in France was met with scepticism and criticism.[4–5] In any event, we continued our work – we managed to stay in front, because no other institution was keen to do UAE. Gradually we became familiar with the advantages of the technique, the good quality of vascular occlusion, and the necrosis that was confined to the myoma preserving the myometrium. We questioned the need for further surgery. Against the advice of younger colleagues, Merland and I decided to abandon immediate surgery and to allow evaluation of the myoma after embolization. In October 1993, we decided to study UAE as the sole treatment of uterine myoma. Embolization of the uterine myoma was born.

The technique was to occlude the distal arteries using polyvinyl alcohol particles of 350–500 μ in size and the proximal branch of the uterine artery using 1–2 mm fragments of a rapidly degradable substance (Curaspon). By the end of 1993, five out of six women had successfully undergone embolization whereas the sixth woman had one of the uterine arteries that could not be catheterized. In 1994, nine more patients were embolized. One of them was complicated by bowel obstruction a week following the procedure necessitating a hysterectomy and bowel resection. This case demonstrated the limitation of the technique.

In 1995, we reported our experience in the *Lancet*.[1] Our report was met with some reservation from two readers who were concerned about the non-comparative and non-randomized nature of the trial, but they recognized our innovative work and the possibilities of improvement. We thank them for their forethought.

A new therapeutic approach was born; we had entered an unknown field and began our work as pioneers.

Worldwide development of uterine artery embolization

Soon after our publication, two medical teams expressed their interest in the technique – the teams from University of California Los Angeles (UCLA) and from Guys Hospital in London. Dr. McLucas from UCLA, who was particularly keen on minimally invasive techniques, while spending time in Paris was the first to contact us. He then introduced this technique in the United States and his team was responsible for the first American publication.[6] The team from London, who had submitted a similar research project to their Ethics Board also visited us and later published their own results.[7]

At the same time, Hutchins and Worthington-Kirsh in Philadelphia, USA, and Sutton, Walker and Forman in Guildford, UK, convinced about the value of the technique, started their own series. Their presentations and publications led to a wider knowledge and technical improvement of UAE.[8,9] Very rapidly, other investigators, especially Pron and Spies, reported their experience and results, contributing to a more extensive knowledge of this method.[10] To date, over 200 papers on UAE have been published, and UAE is in the process of being adopted worldwide.

For the first time, a conservative and minimally invasive technique can avoid a large number of hysterectomies. Hysterectomy is equal to the loss of a very important symbol – the uterus, which gives women the priceless privilege of transmitting life and to which they are naturally and viscerally attached.

I believe that our experience in the embolization of uterine myoma was a beautiful and exceptional adventure. We were lucky to discover something original and significant; our only merit was to have taken advantage of this opportunity.

REFERENCES

1. Ravina JH, Herbreteau D, Cigaru-Vigneron N, et al. (1995). Arterial embolization to treat uterine myomata. *Lancet* **346**: 671–2.

2. Pais SO, Glickman M, Schwartz P, Pingoud E & Berkowitz R (1980). Embolization of pelvic arteries for control of postpartum hemorrhage. *Obstet Gynecol* **55**: 748–8.

3. Sampson JA (1912). The blood supply of uterine myomata. *Surg Gynecol Obstet* **14**: 215–34.

4. Ravina JH, Merland JJ, Herbeteau D, Houdart E, Bouret JM & Madelenat P (1994). Embolization pre-operatoire des fibrome uterins – Resultats preliminaires. *Presse Med* **23**: 1540.

5. Ravina JH, Merland JJ, Ciraru-Vigneron N, Bouret JM, Herbeteau D, Houdart E & Aymard A (1995). Embolization arterielle: un nouveau traitement des menorragies des fibromes uterins. *Presse Med* **25**: 1754.

6. Goodwin SC, Vedantham S, McLucas B, Forno AE & Perella R (1997). Uterine artery embolization for uterine fibroids: results of a pilot study. *J Vasc Interv Radiol* **8**: 517–26.

7. Bradley EA, Reidy JF, Forman RG, Jarosz J & Braude PR (1998). Transcatheter uterine artery embolization to treat large uterine fibroids. *Br J Obstet Gynaecol* **105**: 235–40.

8. Worthington-Kirsch RL, Hutchins FL & Popky PL (1998). Uterine artey embolization for the management of leiomyomas: quality of life assessment and clinical response. *Radiology* **208**: 625–9.

9. Walker W, Green A & Sutton C (1999). Bilateral uterine artery embolization for myoma: results, complications and failures. *Min Invas Ther Allied Technol* **8**: 449–54.

10. Spies JB, Ascher SA, Roth AR, et al. (2001). Uterine artery embolization for leiomyomata. *Obstet Gynecol* **98**: 29–34.

11

Uterine artery embolization – vascular anatomic considerations and procedure techniques

Robert L. Worthington-Kirsch[1] and Linda A. Hughes[2]

[1]Image Guided Surgery Associates, Pennsylvania, USA
[2]Holy Cross Hospital, Florida, USA

Anatomic considerations

Familiarity with the relevant vascular anatomy is absolutely essential before discussion of the uterine artery embolization (UAE) procedure itself. The internal iliac artery typically bifurcates into two divisions. The posterior division typically originates postero-medially and sweeps laterally out of the pelvis. The dominant vessel of the posterior division is the superior gluteal artery. When performing UAE, the posterior division and its branches must be avoided, as inadvertent embolization of these vessels can lead to severe complications such as buttock necrosis and damage to the sciatic nerve.

The anterior division originates anterolaterally and courses caudad from the internal iliac bifurcation. It has a number of important branches. The dominant vessel of the anterior division is the inferior gluteal artery. The main branches of the anterior division (in the female) are the uterine artery, the cystic artery, the vaginal artery, the rectal artery, and the internal pudendal artery.

The uterine artery is usually the first branch of the anterior division. This pattern is seen in just under half of patients.[1] Most of the standard anatomic texts[2,3] describe its origin as antero-medial. Experience has shown that the origin of the uterine artery is just as likely to be antero-lateral as antero-medial. There are two common anatomic variants for the origin of the uterine artery.[1] In about 40% of patients the internal iliac artery trifurcates into the anterior division, posterior division, and the uterine artery. In about 5% of patients the uterine artery

originates from the internal iliac trunk above the bifurcation.

The uterine artery typically originates at an angle of between 45 and 90 degrees off its parent vessel, and bends sharply caudad in the first few centimeters of its course. Its course can be divided into descending, transverse, and ascending segments. The descending segment runs in the pelvic sidewall and lateral margin of the broad ligament to the level of the uterine cervix. The transverse segment courses medially through the base of the broad ligament towards the uterus. At the level of the junction of the cervix with the lower uterine segment the uterine artery turns cephalad and the ascending segment courses along the lateral margin of the uterus towards the fundus. All of these segments vary in tortuosity, ranging from fairly straight to extremely tortuous – sometimes with multiple complete loops.

The ascending segment gives off branches that penetrate the uterine body and run anteriorly and posteriorly along the periphery of the myometrium.[4,5] Radial branches into the deep myometrium arise from these arcuate vessels. There are rich anastomoses within the uterus between the right and left uterine artery distributions.

While it usually originates alone from its parent vessel, in about 10–15% of cases the uterine artery shares a common origin and proximal segment with the cystic artery. In these cases the cystic artery is smaller and straighter than the uterine artery. When this situation is encountered the uterine artery can be catheterized by first advancing the catheter into the cystic artery and pulling back to define the origin of the uterine artery, which can then be entered with a suitably curved guide wire.

There are three other branches of the uterine artery that are important. A branch to the distal ureter has been described arising from the proximal descending segment.[6] Neither of the authors has demonstrated this branch in clinical practice.

The cervico-vaginal branch arises from the mid to distal portion of the transverse segment or the proximal portion of the ascending segment. These branches collateralize with ascending branches of the vaginal artery. There is concern that this vessel provides supply to nerve fibers and other structures in the cervix, which may be important in sexual response and experience. There has been significant debate in recent years over the importance of excluding this vessel from the embolization field. The authors' recommendation is that embolization be performed with the catheter tip beyond the origin of the cervico-vaginal branch, excluding it from embolization, if this is technically feasible. However, in many cases this will not be technically feasible due to vessel tortuosity and/or the location of the branch origin. Including the cervico-vaginal branch in the embolization field is not considered a technical fault.

There is an anastomotic connection between the uterine artery and ovarian artery branches in many women. This is visible on initial injection of the uterine artery in 10–15% of cases.[7] In these cases one must be careful to minimize reflux of embolic particles into the ovarian artery to avoid embolization of the ovary itself. Fortunately, the ovary itself is located several centimeters cephalad to the site of the anastomosis itself and a small amount of "to-and-fro" reflux across the anastomosis does not put the ovary in danger.

There are three anatomic variants, which may be encountered during the course of the catheterization.[8] In about 1% of patients, part or all of the uterine artery is absent. In about 0.3% of patients, both uterine arteries are absent. In these cases the intrauterine vessels are branches of the ovarian artery. In about 0.1% of patients, there is no single uterine artery trunk, but multiple small branches of the internal iliac artery supply the uterus.

Pre-procedure evaluation

Consultation

Before having uterine artery embolization, it is essential that the patient first have a formal consultation with the interventional radiologist. The consultation gives the interventional physician the opportunity to obtain a relevant history, review the necessary imaging, explain the procedure (including its potential risks and complications), and answer any questions that a patient has regarding the procedure. The interventional radiologist is the clinician that evaluates the patient and determines if she is a candidate for the intervention. This is particularly important, as there are many misconceptions and myths regarding the procedure and post procedure convalescence, which can and should be addressed at the time of the consultation. The authors stress the importance during consultation of urging the patient to know and understand her options so that the patient can then make an informed decision.

The issue of future fertility must also be investigated. It is important to know what the patient's future intentions are as well as her desires for potentially preserving fertility. Many women are not interested in future fertility, but rather are interested in avoiding surgery and are seeking a minimally invasive treatment for their symptoms. Review of systems for renal insufficiency, history of pelvic inflammatory disease, and contrast allergies are also critical prior to any planned intervention.

Preoperative studies

Imaging is essential to confirm the diagnosis of fibroids and establish a baseline prior to the procedure. This is to assess the fibroid uterus, including the size, number, and location of fibroids, the presence or absence of pedunculated fibroids, evaluate the endometrium, and exclude any adnexal and/or ovarian pathology. The majority of interventional radiologists use ultrasound and reserve magnetic resonance imaging (MRI) for cases where the ultrasound was incomplete or could not fully evaluate the female pelvis or distinguish a fibroid uterus from adenomyosis. A growing number of physicians, however, are routinely using a targeted limited MRI protocol instead of ultrasound. These studies are viewed in conjunction with the pelvic examination.

A recent Pap (Papanicolaou) smear (less than one year) is required to exclude any significant cervical pathology. There is some debate about the necessity of endometrial evaluation before UAE. If the imaging studies clearly show a normal endometrial canal, no further endometrial evaluation may be necessary. However, in many women with fibroid disease the endometrial canal cannot be fully evaluated by ultrasound or MRI. Evaluation by hysteroscopy, endometrial biopsy, or D&C is often indicated, particularly in women with abnormal bleeding. In the opinion of the authors, the exact method chosen is best left to the discretion of the referring gynecologist. In some patients the uterus is sufficiently distorted that hysteroscopy or endometrial biopsy are not feasible. In our experience the referring gynecologist has usually not felt that the index of suspicion for endometrial pathology is high enough to justify a hysteroscopy or a D&C.

Referral relationships

While uterine embolization is not a new procedure, the application of the technique to fibroid disease is relatively recent and many gynecologists are not familiar with the details of the procedure and consequent patient management issues. Open lines of communication between the interventional radiologist and the gynecologist are critical for proper management of the patient undergoing UAE.

Uterine artery embolization procedure

Patients are admitted the morning of the procedure. The preprocedure routine varies slightly among interventional radiologists but overall is very similar. The authors believe that one of the most critical aspects of a successful UAE is the management of post-procedure pain and nausea. Many clinicians premedicate patients with non-steroidal anti-inflammatory drugs (NSAIDs) either before or during the embolization. Some, including the authors, also use anti-emetic prophylaxis with transdermal scopolamine or metoclopramide.

The protocol prior to the actual procedure includes placement of an IV line, blood work including: coagulation profile, complete blood count (CBC), blood urea nitrogen (BUN), creatinine, follicular stimulating hormone (FSH), and a pregnancy test. All patients are given a dose of intravenous antibiotics (the exact medication and dose varies depending upon physician and patient allergy history).

Many clinicians, including the authors, have a Foley catheter inserted prior to the procedure. This serves two purposes. First and foremost, it keeps the urinary bladder empty of the contrast which collects during the procedure and can obscure visualization of the fibroid blood supply. This also reduces the radiation dose from the procedure. Secondly, unless a closure device is used, patients are at bed rest for five to six hours after the procedure to allow time for the arteriotomy to heal. The Foley catheter allows the bladder to be drained during this time, greatly improving patient comfort.

One of the advantages of UAE is the fact that it is a minimally invasive procedure, which is routinely performed without the need for general anesthesia. Most interventional radiologists use a combination of narcotics and benzodiazepines for conscious sedation,[9–11] however there are some physicians who use spinal analgesia.

The embolization procedure can be performed from either a unilateral or bilateral approach. Most interventional radiologists use a right unilateral approach. Patients typically receive antibiotic and antiemetic prophylaxis before the procedure.[9–12]

Mapping injections are used to define the individual anatomy (Figures 11.1–11.3)[a]. Most clinicians catheterize the contralateral (left) internal iliac artery first, although some prefer to treat the larger of the

---

[a] Figures 11.3–11.6 are all from the same patient. Figures 11.7–11.9 are from another patient. All other Figures are from different patients.

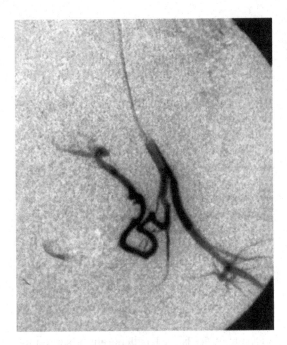

Figure 11.1. Injection of the left internal iliac artery showing typical appearance of the origin of the uterine artery. Courtesy of Robert L. Worthington-Kirsch.

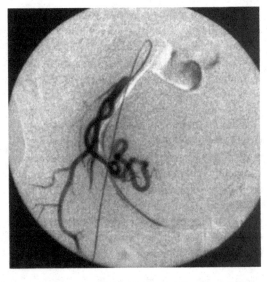

Figure 11.2. Injection of the right internal iliac artery showing typical appearance of the origin of the uterine artery. Courtesy of Robert L. Worthington-Kirsch.

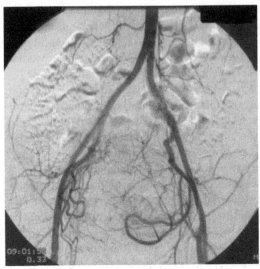

Figure 11.3. Pre-embolization mapping arteriogram of the pelvis showing both uterine arteries and their branches in the uterus. Courtesy of Linda A. Hughes.

two uterine arteries first, expecting flow redistribution after the first embolization to cause dilation of the smaller uterine artery.[13] In any case, once the specific anatomy of the target vessel is defined, the uterine artery is catheterized. If large enough, the uterine artery is catheterized with a standard 4 or 5 French size end-hole visceral catheter. If the vessel is small, extremely tortuous, or shows evidence of spasm, a microcatheter can be advanced through the standard catheter for the embolization. The catheter tip should ideally be positioned in the transverse segment of the uterine artery, distal to the origin of the cervico-vaginal branch (as discussed above).

Once the catheter is in place, an arteriogram of the uterine artery is performed to evaluate the distribution and speed of flow, demonstrate any utero-ovarian collaterals, and to exclude any unusual occurrences such as an arterio-venous malformation of the uterus. The embolization can then be performed (Figures 11.4–11.8).

There are three embolic materials currently used for UAE: gelatin sponge, polyvinyl alcohol (PVA) powder, and calibrated tris-acryl microspheres. The majority of the published experience is with PVA

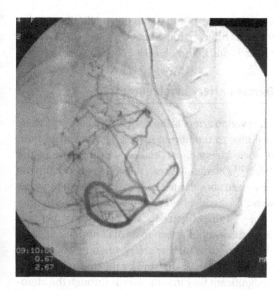

Figure 11.4. Pre-embolization selective injection of the left uterine artery showing typical branching of vessels around the fibroids. Courtesy of Linda A. Hughes.

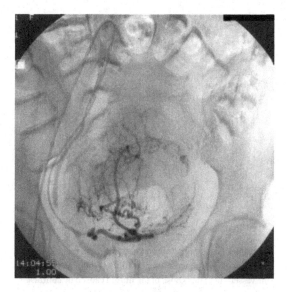

Figure 11.6. Pre-embolization selective injection of the right uterine artery showing typical branching of vessels around the fibroids. Courtesy of Linda A. Hughes.

embolizations, although calibrated microspheres appear to be growing in popularity because they are somewhat easier to use. Gelatin sponge is used rarely, and there is some controversy as to whether or not it should be used for this application. There are currently no published data showing that any specific embolizant is more effective or has a better safety profile than the others.

The embolic material is suspended in dilute contrast and injected into the uterine artery. It is carried into the uterus by blood flow and causes occlusion of the vessels by a combination of physical occlusion and thrombus formation.

Embolic material is injected into the uterine artery until the desired arteriographic endpoint is reached. When UAE was first introduced, embolization was performed to the point of complete occlusion of the uterine artery. Many clinicians now perform a less extensive embolization, using an endpoint of slow flow in the ascending branch of the uterine artery with non-filling of penetrating branches.

After the first uterine artery has been embolized, the other uterine artery is then selectively catheterized and embolized in the same fashion. The

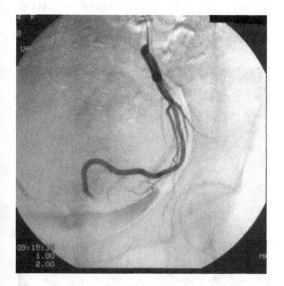

Figure 11.5. Post-embolization injection of the left uterine artery showing absence of flow beyond the main segment of the vessel. Courtesy of Linda A. Hughes.

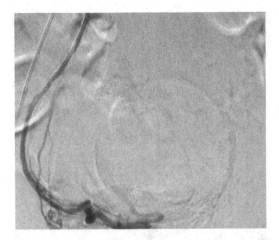

Figure 11.7. Post-embolization injection of the right uterine artery showing absence of flow beyond the main segment of the vessel – note the 'ghost' of the fibroid caused by contrast retention in the tissues after embolization. Courtesy of Linda A. Hughes.

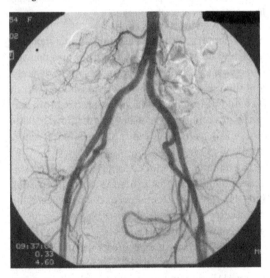

Figure 11.8. Post uterine artery embolization mapping arteriogram showing absence of flow into the branches of the uterine arteries. Courtesy of Linda A. Hughes.

procedure is then completed and the patient transferred to a room or recovery area. Patients are discharged on either the same day or after an overnight stay. Discharge medications are similar to those used for management of patients who have had

a spontaneous fibroid infarction – NSAIDs supplemented with narcotics as needed. Recovery is rapid, typically one to three weeks.

Ovarian artery involvement

The ovarian artery is the most likely source of collateral flow to the fibroid uterus. This collateral flow, if not addressed, can cause clinical failure of the UAE.[8,14] Ovarian flow can take one of two forms. As discussed above, in about 1% of cases anatomic variants occur with absence of part or all of the uterine artery. In these instances the flow to the uterus is from the ovarian artery. In a small number of cases there is normal uterine artery anatomy but there is sufficient vascular demand by the uterus that there is significant flow into the uterus through the utero-ovarian collateral. This is visible in about 5% of cases (Figures 11.9 & 11.10).

When the ovarian artery provides supplemental flow to the uterus, it is important to ensure that sufficient embolic material gets to the portions of the uterine fundus beyond the point of ovarian artery

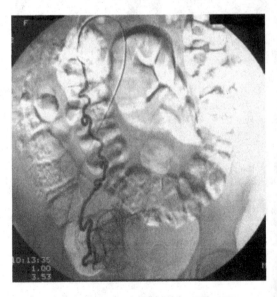

Figure 11.9. Selective injection of the right ovarian artery (arising directly from the aorta) showing branches into the uterus supplying fibroids in the region of the fundus. Courtesy of Linda A. Hughes.

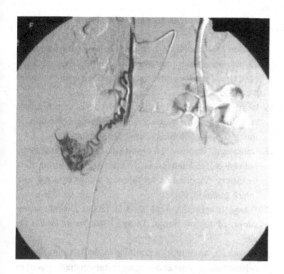

Figure 11.10. Selective injection of the right ovarian artery (arising directly from the aorta) showing supply only to the ovary without branches to the uterus – note how the pattern of perfusion outlines the ovarian follicles. Courtesy of Linda A. Hughes.

inflow. Careful monitoring of the injection pressure during embolization will ensure that there is minimal reflux across the anastomosis and that embolic material does get beyond the anastomosis. Allowing a small amount of reflux (no more than a centimeter or so) and then having the refluxed material wash back into the uterus can ensure that the ovarian artery inflow helps to carry embolic material into the fundus, without embolizing the ovary itself, which is found several centimeters proximal to the utero-ovarian anastomosis.

When an anatomic variant of the uterine artery is observed, or if a portion of the uterus isn't demonstrated during embolization of the uterine arteries, then selective injection of the ovarian artery on the relevant side may be useful.

The orifice of the left ovarian artery is usually found arising from the aorta inferior and medial to the orifice of the left renal artery. The right ovarian artery is most often found arising from the aorta distal to and slightly to the right of the orifice of the superior mesenteric artery.

When the ovarian artery is selected and injection shows that there is flow to the uterus, embolization can be considered. Care should be taken to avoid an embolization scheme, which risks embolization of the ovary itself. Proximal embolization of the ovarian artery with relatively large gelatin sponge pledgets can cut the filling pressure into the uterus enough to ensure a good clinical result from the embolization without endangering the ovaries.[15] Embolization of the ovarian artery with relatively large particles (over 500–600µ) can also be considered because these particles are likely to be too large to enter the ovarian vascular bed and so will bypass the ovary and go into the uterine vascular bed.[16,17]

Some authors have advocated routine pre-embolization aortography to assess the ovarian arteries.[18] However, the authors feel that this is unnecessary. It is important to do this *after* the uterine arteries have been embolized because embolization of the uterine arteries may well have already occluded any intrauterine branches, which the ovarian artery was supplying. It is still unknown whether or not aortography should be performed routinely after embolization of the uterine arteries. The authors only do so when they suspect a residual ovarian artery contribution after the uterine arteries have been embolized.

REFERENCES

1. Gomez-Jorge J, Kuyoung A & Spies JB (2000). Uterine artery anatomy relevant to uterine leiomyomata embolization. Abstract presented at *SCVIR Uterine Artery Embolization (UAE) Conference, 14 October 2000, Washington, DC.*
2. Netter FH (1954). *The CIBA Collection of Medical Illustrations*, vol. 2, *Reproductive System*, pp. 97–9. Summit, NJ: Ciba Pharmaceuticals.
3. Merland JJ & Chiras J (1981). *Arteriography of the Pelvis*, pp. 13–14. New York: Springer Verlag.
4. Sampson JA (1912). The blood supply of uterine myomata. *Surg Gynecol Obstet* 14: 215–34.
5. Fernstrom I (1955). Arteriography of the uterine artery. *Acta Radiologica* 122(Suppl): 21–8.
6. Kadir S (1991). *Atlas of Normal and Variant Angiographic Anatomy*, p. 279. Philadelphia: WB Saunders.
7. Pelage JP, LeDref O, Soyer P, et al. (1999). Arterial anatomy of the female genital tract: variations and relevance to transcatheter embolization of the uterus. *Am J Roentgenol* 172: 989–44.

8. Worthington-Kirsch RL, Walker WJ, Adler L & Hutchins FL (1999). Anatomic variation in the uterine arteries: a cause of failure of uterine artery embolisation for the management of symptomatic fibroids. *Min Invas Ther & Allied Technol* **8**: 425–527.

9. Goodwin SC, Vedantham S, McLucas B, Forno AE & Perella R (1997). Uterine artery embolization for uterine fibroids: results of a pilot study. *J Vasc Interv Radiol* **8**: 517–26.

10. Worthington-Kirsch RL, Hutchins FL & Popky PL (1998). Uterine artery embolization for the management of leiomyomas: quality of life assessment and clinical response. *Radiology* **208**: 625–9.

11. Spies JB, Scialli AR, Jha RC, et al. (1999). Initial results from uterine artery embolization for symptomatic leiomyomata. *J Vasc Interv Radiol* **10**: 1149–57.

12. Worthington-Kirsch RL, Roberts AC & Hughes LA. Antiemetic prophylaxis for uterine artery embolization for the treatment for fibroids. (Unpublished data.)

13. Worthington-Kirsch RL (1999). Flow redistribution during uterine artery embolization for the management of symptomatic fibroids. (Letter.) *J Vasc Interv Radiol* **10**(2): 237–8.

14. Matson M, Nicholson A & Belli AM (2000). Anastamoses of the ovarian and uterine arteries: a potential pitfall and cause of failure of uterine embolization. *Cardiovasc Interv Radiol* **23**: 393–6.

15. Worthington-Kirsch RL. Safety and efficacy of ovarian artery embolization in the course of uterine artery embolization for the treatment of fibroids. (Unpublished data.)

16. Andrews RT, Bromley PJ & Pfister ME (2000). Successful embolization of collaterals from the ovarian artery during uterine artery embolization for fibroids: a case report. *J Vasc Interv Radiol* **11**: 607–10.

17. Pelage JP, LeDref O, Jacob D, et al. (2000). Ovarian artery supply of uterine fibroid. (Letter.) *J Vasc Interv Radiol* **11**: 535.

18. Binkert CA, Andrews RT & Kaufman JA (2001). Utility of nonselective abdominal aortography in demonstrating ovarian artery collaterals in patients undergoing uterine artery embolization for fibroids. *J Vasc Interv Radiol* **12**: 841–5.

12

Pain management during and after uterine artery embolization

Suresh Vedantham[1] and Scott C. Goodwin[2]

[1]Washington University in St. Louis, Missouri, USA
[2]Veteran Administration, UCLA Medical Center, California, USA

Introduction

Uterine artery embolization (UAE) has evolved into a safe and effective alternative treatment for women with symptomatic uterine fibroids. Published series have documented clinical response rates of 81–94% for menorrhagia and 64–96% for bulk-related symptoms, with high patient satisfaction ratings and few major complications.[1–9] The advantages of this procedure include shorter hospitalizations, uterine preservation, and the ability to treat all myomata in the uterus in a single session. Importantly, the non-surgical nature of UAE enables the procedure to be performed under conscious sedation, a very important advantage that significantly lowers the risks and morbidity of the procedure.

Many critical aspects of establishing a UAE program relate to ensuring the tolerability of the procedure. Careful attention to compassionate peri-procedural patient care is paramount in encouraging physicians to continue recommending this treatment option to their patients. With the UAE patient population, many referrals reach the interventionalist through word-of-mouth patient-to-patient referral; the practitioner who does not expend maximum effort ensuring patient comfort will very rightly not receive such referrals. The interventional physician must be able to provide the patient with reasonable expectations about the peri-procedural discomfort she might encounter, establish a routine monitoring and sedation plan for UAE, ensure a suitable environment for post-procedure patient recovery, prevent and treat post-procedural symptoms, communicate with the patient and nursing staff, and monitor patient satisfaction.

Developing a pain management system: principles

Nearly all patients experience pelvic pain following UAE, but there exists tremendous variation in the amount and duration of post-procedural symptoms. Some investigators have theorized that the amount of peri-procedural pain may correlate with pre-procedural uterine size, but the existing data does not support this conclusion.[10] At this time, no reliable method exists to predict which patients will experience more peri-procedural discomfort than others. Similarly, there is no relationship between the amount of post-procedural pain experienced and the clinical response to UAE.[10]

In devising a method of addressing the anesthetic requirements of the UAE procedure and those of the post-procedural period, interventionalists who take the time to pro-actively and systematically address several key aspects of patient management will likely have the greatest success: (1) be familiar with the expected amount and time course of pain after UAE, and understand which controllable intra-procedural factors may influence post-procedural symptoms; (2) understand which deviations from the usual pattern should raise suspicion for potential complications of UAE, and convey this understanding to the patient; (3) develop a pain management protocol for the procedure, the in-hospital post-procedure period, and the outpatient recovery period, incorporating anesthesiologist expertise in this process if possible. In designing a medication regimen, remember to address common associated symptoms such as nausea, vomiting, constipation, and fever; (4) ensure that the patient and her nurse have continuous access to an interventional radiology physician to manage any breakthrough pain; and (5) solicit feedback regarding the success of the pain regimen and overall patient satisfaction with the UAE experience. While significant variation exists from institution to institution, the following sections describe the most common approaches to ensuring patient comfort during and after UAE.

Patient comfort during the UAE procedure

While the earliest UAE patients were treated under general anesthesia, most interventionalists currently believe that moderate conscious sedation achieves the optimal combination of maximum safety and patient comfort.[11,12] The American Society of Anesthesiologists (ASA) guidelines define conscious sedation as "a drug-induced depression of consciousness during which patients respond purposefully to verbal commands, either alone or accompanied by light tactile stimulation. No interventions are required to maintain a patent airway, and spontaneous ventilation is adequate. Cardiovascular function is usually maintained." Per ASA guidelines, patients must undergo detailed pre-sedation evaluation and must refrain from ingesting solid foods (six to eight hours) or clear liquids (two to three hours) before the procedure. Patients must be monitored for level of consciousness, ventilation, oxygenation, and cardiovascular vital signs during and after the procedure.[13] This evaluation and monitoring capability is currently standard in most interventional radiology practice settings.

The UAE procedure itself is almost always well-tolerated by the patient. There are typically two time points in the UAE procedure when the patient may feel some discomfort. First, minor pain may be encountered during femoral arterial access. This can be minimized through adequate sedation and by locally administering a small amount of 1% lidocaine into the groin just prior to femoral arterial puncture, as is standard for any arteriographic procedure. After this point, the patient will feel little or no discomfort until the end of the UAE procedure. However, after the second uterine artery is embolized, significant pelvic pain may begin. This pain is usually described as heavy, crampy pain similar to but more pronounced than menstrual cramping. Fever, nausea, vomiting, and/or weakness, as observed after other organ embolizations, often accompany the pain. The usual pattern is for pain to start during or soon after the UAE procedure, to peak 6–12 hours after the procedure, and to gradually subside over a period of 12 hours to several days. The pain peak can be delayed by 12–24 hours, and rarely by more than one day. These symptoms are thought to result from infarction of the uterine fibroids, with release of tissue breakdown products by the degenerating tissue.[14]

Pain management protocols differ significantly in various institutions where UAE is performed. A sample protocol is presented in Table 12.1. Most practitioners arrange for the patient to arrive in the department in the early morning. At that time, an intravenous line is placed, the pre-sedation work-up is completed, and anxiolytic medications can be administered to nervous patients before entering the procedure room. Medication regimens for UAE have evolved to include several important elements: (1) an intravenous opioid analgesic agent, usually fentanyl or morphine; (2) a short-acting anxiolytic/sedative agent, usually a benzodiazepine such as midazolam; (3) a parenteral non-steroidal anti-inflammatory drug (NSAID) such as ketorolac has become standard for UAE pain management, because the character of post-UAE pain has so much in common with other causes of uterine pain. While the use of NSAID-containing regimens has not been scientifically compared with regimens not incorporating NSAIDs, some investigators have noticed significant improvements in the tolerability of UAE after the addition of NSAIDs. In our institution, two 30 mg doses of ketorolac are administered parenterally, the first

Table 12.1. Sample protocol for uterine artery embolization pain management

Pre-procedure holding area
Ketorolac 30 mg IV × 1 dose
Midazolam 1–2 mg IV × 1 dose (optional)

Procedural medications (must maintain oxygen saturation > 92% and SBP > 90 mmHg)
Throughout UAE procedure:
Fentanyl 50–75 μg IV × 1 dose then 25–50 μg IV every
 10 minutes as needed
Midazolam 1–2 mg IV × 1 dose then 0.5–1.0 mg IV every
 10 minutes as needed

After the first uterine artery has been embolized:
Ketorolac 30 mg IV × 1 dose
Ondansetron 4 mg IV × 1 dose

After the second uterine artery has been embolized:
Fentanyl 50 μg IV × 1 dose
Morphine 3 mg IV × 1 dose
Midazolam 1.0 mg × 1 dose

Post-procedure in-house medications
Day of procedure:
Morphine PCA Pump (2 mg doses, 10 minute lockout)
Ketorolac 30 mg IV every 6 hours until next morning
Ondansetron 4 mg IV every 8 hours until next morning
Acetaminophen 650 mg po every 6 hours

When patient feels ready to switch to oral medications (usually
 the morning after UAE):
Hydrocodone 10 mg po every 6 hours
Acetaminophen 1000 mg po every 6 hours
Ibuprofen 600 mg po every 8 hours
Ondansetron 4 mg po every 8 hours

Always available for breakthrough symptoms:
Morphine 3–5 mg IV every 3 hours as needed for pain
Ondansetron 4 mg IV every 8 hours as needed for nausea
Prochlorperazine 10 mg IV every 6 hours as needed for nausea
Call IR physician if these medications are not sufficient!

IR: interventional radiology.

in the pre-procedure holding area and the second after embolization of the first uterine artery has been completed; (4) a strong anti-emetic – in our practice, we administer a single dose of ondansetron during the procedure, although nausea (when it occurs)

does not typically occur until after the procedure. With this combination, patients will be comfortable during the vast majority of UAE procedures.

A few controllable procedural factors may influence the amount of peri-procedural discomfort to the patient, but the relative importance of each factor upon peri-procedural pain has not yet been fully characterized. Some investigators have attempted to use routine intra-arterial administration of preservative-free, 1% lidocaine to reduce the pain caused by UAE, based on prior studies in which intra-arterial lidocaine was successful in controlling pain caused by contrast material injection and hepatic chemoembolization.[15,16] In one controlled study, patients receiving intra-arterial lidocaine experienced less subjective pain, although analgesic medication requirements were not altered. Unfortunately, moderate to severe vasospasm occurred in most patients receiving lidocaine, hampering the ability to embolize the uterine arteries. For this reason, the investigators did not recommend this method for pain control.[17]

Many have speculated that the arterial level and completeness of embolization may correlate with the amount of peri-procedural pain after UAE. In this respect, two controllable factors are the embolic agent chosen and the angiographic endpoint of embolization. While Gelfoam, calibrated microspheres, and polyvinyl alcohol particles (PVA) of various sizes have all been utilized for UAE, only one study has directly addressed the success rates and tolerability of UAE when using the different agents.[18–20] In this study of 72 patients undergoing UAE with either PVA or calibrated microspheres (Embospheres, Biosphere Medical, Rockland, MA), no difference in subjective pain scores or the amount of analgesic agent used was observed.[20] No systematic comparison has yet been performed to evaluate the optimal angiographic endpoint for embolization. As more experience has been gained with UAE, it has become clear that embolizing each uterine artery to complete stasis is not necessary, and many have evolved towards terminating embolization when slow flow in the ascending uterine artery segment is observed. It will be interesting to learn whether the amount of peri-procedural pain is influenced by this change in technique. Clearly, the questions regarding the influence of embolic agent choice and angiographic endpoint upon peri-procedural symptoms will need to be addressed in prospective studies.

The use of percutaneous femoral arterial closure devices after angiographic procedures permits early post-procedure ambulation.[21] As such, some interventionalists use these devices routinely in UAE patients to improve patient comfort by allowing earlier ambulation and mobility. Many others prefer to reserve this option for patients with significant pre-procedure back pain or other problems that make prolonged post-procedure bedrest painful or difficult.

Post-procedural pain management

Because the onset of crampy pain often immediately follows embolization of the second uterine artery, pain management protocols need to be planned prospectively. To ensure patient comfort during the transition from the procedure room to the post-procedure observation area, we and others typically administer significant bolus doses of analgesic and sedative medications just prior to removing the patient from the angiography suite. If a patient-controlled analgesia (PCA) pump is being used, it is important to train the patient in its use before the procedure, and to have the pump ready by the end of the procedure.

Because pain after UAE usually peaks 6–12 hours after the procedure, most investigators choose to observe UAE patients in the hospital overnight. The patient is allowed a light dinner (if she desires), and may ambulate four to six hours after the procedure (or sooner if a percutaneous closure device has been utilized). Many of the same elements that are used for intra-procedural sedation are continued during the post-procedure phase. The specific elements of the post-procedural pain regimen should include: (1) an opioid analgesic; (2) an NSAID; (3) a strong anti-emetic medication; (4) a laxative, since opioid narcotics may cause constipation; and (5) an

anti-pyretic agent, since fevers may continue for several days after UAE.

We believe that patient-controlled analgesia provides the best method of pain relief in the post-procedure period. This method of drug administration eliminates the delays inherent in conveying a request for pain medications to the nurse and physician, and in procuring the dose. Each hospital has its own policy for arranging for a PCA pump, with some hospitals requiring consultation with an anesthesiologist. Any one of several agents can be administered via the pump, including morphine, hydromorphone, and meperidine. When using a PCA pump, it is important to write orders for medications to treat breakthrough pain. The evening of the procedure, the interventionalist should reinforce an awareness of the patient's analgesia needs with her nurse, and encourage him/her to contact the interventional radiology physician if the analgesic regimen is not effective. If the interventionalist cannot control breakthrough pain expeditiously, early consultation of a pain specialist from the anesthesiology department should be obtained.

The PCA pump is discontinued when the patient feels ready – in most cases, this occurs the morning after the procedure. The patient is switched to oral opioid and NSAID medications, although intravenous opioids are still available upon request. The patient is encouraged to eat, drink, and ambulate a little. This period in essence serves as a six-hour test of the patient's ability to maintain herself at home. If the patient is able to ambulate and eat lunch without difficulty, she is discharged with prescriptions for oral analgesics, anti-emetics, anti-pyretics, and a stool softener. A sample discharge medications protocol is presented in Table 12.2. The patient is given contact information for the interventional radiology physician and/or nurse coordinator. She is instructed to taper her analgesics as tolerated over the next several days, and to maintain anti-pyretic therapy for five days. Nearly all patients feel well enough to be discharged the day after the procedure, with a small minority requiring a second night in the hospital. During the first week we maintain close telephone contact with UAE patients to make sure they

Table 12.2. Sample discharge medications after uterine artery embolization

Discharge medications
Hydrocodone 5–10 mg po every 6 hours for one day then as needed for pain
Ondansetron 4 mg tablet po every 8 hours for one day then as needed for nausea
Ibuprofen 600 mg po every 8 hours for three days then as needed for pain
Acetaminophen 650 mg po every 6 hours for five days
Prochlorperazine 10 mg po every 6 hours as needed for nausea
Colace 10 mg po every 12 hours as needed for constipation
Call IR physician if these medications are not sufficient!

IR: interventional radiology.

are progressing appropriately. Most patients will be back to normal function in 14 days.

Patients are informed that increasing pelvic pain more than three days after the procedure and fevers more than five days after the procedure should prompt a telephone call to the interventionalist, as they might represent early signs of infection. A small percentage of UAE patients (2–10%) will require re-admission to the hospital for post-embolization syndrome, characterized by fever, nausea, vomiting, and pain that occurs several days to two weeks after the procedure.[3,9] These patients are usually admit-ted, hydrated, and treated for pain for one to two days. The symptoms generally improve rapidly. If symptoms continue, evaluation for possible infec-tion is undertaken and the patient is placed on intravenous antibiotics. The incidence of uterine infection after UAE is actually quite small, with most such patients treated successfully with antibi-otics.

The patient is also made aware that a small per-centage of UAE patients can slough fibroids. While this usually causes passing discomfort, occasion-ally a sloughed fibroid will impact at the cervix and cause significant persistent cramping.[22,23] Because such patients may be slightly more prone to infec-tion, close follow-up is essential. In most cases, the fibroid will pass spontaneously; if this does not occur

or if the patient's symptoms are acute, the fibroid can be removed hysteroscopically.

Outpatient UAE

The idea of outpatient UAE is an attractive one, and the observation that at least some UAE patients can be discharged the evening of the procedure has been made by several investigators.[3,9] The main advantage of staying in a hospital setting overnight is the ability to receive continuous nursing care and intravenous analgesics. The main advantage of being discharged is a more comfortable home environment, providing a helpful responsible adult is available to assist the patient.

At least one group has actively investigated the possibility of devising an aggressive medication and patient surveillance protocol to follow outpatient UAE. In one published study of 47 patients undergo-ing outpatient UAE, patient satisfaction with same-day discharge after UAE was 94%, with more than 90% reporting that oral medications were success-ful in controlling their symptoms.[8] In this study, a careful protocol of defined telephone follow-up, staff availability, and oral medications was followed. Hence, under the proper conditions, selected pa-tients may be successfully treated with an outpatient approach.

Conclusion

Uterine fibroid embolization has proven to be a well-tolerated, minimally invasive treatment for symp-tomatic uterine fibroids, and is routinely performed using conscious sedation. The combination of opi-oid and NSAID analgesics is effective for intra-procedural and post-procedural pain management, with additional benzodiazepine sedation/anxiolysis for the procedure itself. Nearly all patients can be discharged the day after the procedure, and some evolution towards performing UAE as an outpa-tient procedure is occurring. With a systematic, pro-active approach to peri-procedural pain control, health care team education, and patient education, excellent results can be achieved in terms of patient comfort and overall satisfaction with the UAE procedure.

REFERENCES

1. Andersen PE, Lund N, Justesen P, et al. (2001). Uterine artery embolization for symptomatic uterine fibroids: initial success and short-term results. *Acta Radiol* **42**: 234–8.
2. Brunereau L, Herbreteau D, Gallas S, et al. (2000). Uterine artery embolization in the primary treatment of uterine leiomyomas: technical features and prospective follow-up with clinical and sonographic examination in 58 patients. *Am J Roentgenol* **175**: 1267–72.
3. Goodwin S, McLucas B, Lee M, et al. (1999). Uterine artery embolization for the treatment of uterine leiomyomata: midterm results. *J Vasc Interv Radiol* **10**: 1159–65.
4. Hutchins F, Worthington-Kirsch R & Berkowitz R (1999). Selective uterine artery embolization as primary treatment for symptomatic leiomyomata uteri. *J Am Assoc Gynecol Laparosc* **6**: 279–84.
5. McLucas B, Adler L & Perella R (2001). Uterine fibroid embolization: nonsurgical treatment for symptomatic fibroids. *J Am Coll Surg* **192**: 95–105.
6. Pelage J, LeDref O, Soyer P, et al. (2000). Fibroid-related menorrhagia: treatment with superselective embolization of the uterine arteries and midterm follow-up. *Radiology* **215**: 428–31.
7. Ravina J, Cicaru-Vigneron N, Aymard A, et al. (1999). Uterine artery embolisation for fibroid disease: results of a 6 year study. *Min Invas Ther Allied Technol* **8**: 441–7.
8. Siskin G, Stainken B, Dowling K, et al. (2000). Outpatient uterine artery embolization for symptomatic uterine fibroids: experience in 49 patients. *J Vasc Interv Radiol* **11**: 305–11.
9. Spies J, Ascher SA, Roth AR, et al. (2001). Uterine artery embolization for leiomyomata. *Obstet Gynecol* **98**: 29–34.
10. Roth AR, Spies JB, Walsh SM, et al. (2000). Pain after uterine artery embolization for leiomyomata: can its severity be predicted and does severity predict outcome? *J Vasc Interv Radiol* **11**: 1047–52.
11. Goodwin SC, Vedantham S, McLucas B, et al. (1997). Preliminary experience with uterine artery embolization for uterine fibroids. *J Vasc Interv Radiol* **8**: 517–26.
12. Ravina J, Herbreteau D, Ciraru-Vigneron N, et al. (1995). Arterial embolisation to treat uterine myomata. *Lancet* **346**: 671–2.
13. American Society of Anesthesiologists Task Force on Sedation and Analgesia by Non-Anesthesiologists (2002). Practice guidelines for sedation and analgesia by non-anesthesiologists. *Anesthesiology* **96**(4): 1004–17.
14. Lipman JC (2002). UAE: post-procedure management and complications. *J Vasc Interv Radiol* Suppl **13**(2, Pt 2): P242–P244.
15. Wildrich WC, Singer RJ, Robbins AH, et al. (1977). The use of intra-arterial lidocaine to control pain due to aortofemoral arteriography. *Radiology* **124**: 37–41.
16. Molgaard CP, Teitelbaum GP, Pentecost MJ, et al. (1990). Intraarterial administration of lidocaine for analgesia in hepatic chemoembolization. *J Vasc Interv Radiol* **1**: 81–5.
17. Keyoung JA, Levy EB, Roth AR, et al. (2001). Intraarterial lidocaine for pain control after uterine artery embolization for leiomyomata. *J Vasc Interv Radiol* **12**: 1065–9.
18. Katsumori T, Nakajima K, Mihara T, et al. (2002). Uterine artery embolization using gelatin sponge particles alone for symptomatic uterine fibroids. *Am J Roentgenol* **178**: 135–9.
19. Spies JB, Benenati JF, Worthington-Kirsch RL, et al. (2001). Initial experience with use of tris-acryl gelatin microspheres for uterine artery embolization for leiomyomata. *J Vasc Interv Radiol* **12**(9): 1059–63.
20. Ryu RK, Omary RA, Chrisman HB, et al. (2002). Tris-acryl gelatin microspheres versus polyvinyl alcohol particles for uterine artery embolization. (Abstract.) *J Vasc Interv Radiol* Suppl **13**(2, Pt 2): S18.
21. Sanders GJ & Hovsepian DM (2001). Vascular closure devices. In SCVIR Peripheral Vascular Interventions Syllabus, 2nd edn, Darcy MD, Vedantham S, Kaufman J (eds.), pp. 91–98. Fairfax, VA: Society of Cardiovascular and Interventional Radiology.
22. Bradley EA, Reidy JF, Forman RG, et al. (1998). Transcatheter uterine artery embolisation to treat large uterine fibroids. *Br J Obstet Gynecol* **105**: 235–40.
23. Abbara S, Spies JB, Scialli AR, et al. (1999). Transcervical expulsion of a fibroid as a result of uterine artery embolization for leiomyomata. *J Vasc Interv Radiol* **10**: 409–11.

13

Patient selection, indications, and contraindications

Francis L. Hutchins, Jr.

Annapolis, Maryland, USA

One of the great dilemmas in the utilization of uterine artery embolization (UAE) in the management of fibroids has been the issue of appropriate patient selection. Up to the present time, no well-defined list of indications has been developed. Since this treatment has such a dramatic impact on fibroids, it may be assumed that any woman with symptomatic fibroids is a candidate for this procedure. It was this kind of thinking that resulted in the liberal, routine use of hysterectomy by some.

In viewing the topic of patient selection, a key factor to keep in mind is the role of the patient. It is not sufficient to weigh only the medical indications and contraindications. Especially when the female reproductive organs are involved, the wishes and aspirations of the woman are paramount. In that regard, not only the physician's desire to avoid the hazards of surgery but also the desire of women to avoid uterine surgery has influenced patient selection from the outset (Table 13.1).

More ideal candidates would be the group of women for whom UAE can solve therapeutic problems heretofore unsolvable or provide a better solution (Table 13.2). Patients with substantial health problems such as morbid obesity, diabetes, hypertension, etc, constitute one obvious group. These patients can be very poor candidates for anesthesia and major surgery whereas they pose no contraindication to embolotherapy.[1]

Ravina,[2] in his initial report, substantiated that UAE can be satisfactorily used as a preoperative treatment for patients scheduled for myomectomy. Thus, one can use UAE as a preoperative treatment in women with very large uteri much as use gonadotropin-releasing hormone agonists (GnRHa) to reduce uterine size, intra-operative blood loss, and correct anemia.[3-5] As experienced by Ravina,[6] many women, even with extremely large tumors, will find their fibroid symptoms satisfactorily addressed and feel they no longer require surgery.[2] It has been observed that the percent reduction in size experienced in very large fibroid uteri (>1000 cc) is greater then in smaller uteri.[7] Thus UAE can be utilized to triage women with very large uteri to surgery or no surgery (Figure 13.1). In this algorithm, three to six months after embolization women can be assessed for their need for further treatment. Those with persistent symptoms can be offered surgery. Those with satisfactory improvement or ablation of their symptoms need no further therapy.

Patients who will not accept transfusion are also excellent candidates for UAE. This non-surgical alternative with low risk for significant blood loss or complications[8] is a benefit to both patient and surgeon. Another option is to perform surgery after UAE in a way similar to GnRHa to correct anemia and reduce the risk of intra-operative blood loss.

Several years ago, in our center in Philadelphia, we saw a patient with intractable life threatening menorrhagia. The young woman had been treated with hormone therapy and transfusions over several months. Prior to transfer, she had been hospitalized for another severe episode of bleeding that failed to respond to any treatment. Hysterectomy was considered. This was especially undesirable because the young woman was desirous of pregnancy.

Table 13.1. Indications for uterine artery embolization

- Symptomatic fibroids – bleeding, pressure, infertility (?), etc.
- Desire to avoid surgery??

Table 13.2. Ideal indications

- Poor surgical candidates
- Preop or primary treatment for excessively large uterus
- When transfusion not acceptable
- Acute intractable hemorhage from fibroids

Table 13.3. Less ideal candidates

- Small uterus (<600 cc) and single tumor
- Single resectable submucous fibroid
- Candidates for endometrial ablation?

Table 13.4. Contraindications to uterine artery embolization

- Pregnancy
- Menopause
- Severe contrast allergy
- Renal failure
- A–V malformation
- Unknown pelvic mass

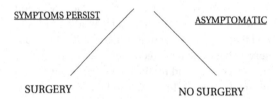

OPTIONS AFTER UAE

Figure 13.1. Uterine artery embolization (UAE) algorithm.

It was inquired as to whether UAE could be tried. We agreed and performed the procedure on an emergency basis. There was dramatic cessation of the menorrhagia. Subsequently, she was found to have a submucous fibroid that was resected. She eventually conceived with IVF and delivered healthy twins at term.

This was an unusual occurrence but demonstrated a unique application of embolotherapy. Although not frequent, such situations do occur from time-to-time when other conservative therapies seem to be ineffective. Of particular note is the fact that embolization has long been used as an emergency treatment for pelvic hemorrhage of many causes including: molar pregnancy, postpartum hemorrhage and pelvic cancer.[9–10] This just represents another variation.

As with all therapies, there are some women with fibroids for whom UAE though feasible is less than ideal (Table 13.3). These include mainly women who could be easily treated with other modalities. Women with a single fundal fibroid that could be easily removed by laparoscopy or by minilaparotomy arguably may also fall into this category.

More obvious is the woman who has a single small submucous fibroid that is easily resected especially if she is desirous of endometrial ablation. The ease and safety with which resectoscopic surgery can be performed by experienced individuals makes it superior to UAE for most patients with limited but highly symptomatic disease.

Contraindications

There are few contraindications to embolotherapy for fibroids (Table 13.4) and they infrequently arise. It is nevertheless important to review them with the intent of giving an overview, as well as adding specific concerns of the gynecologist in prescribing UAE for the treatment of leiomyomata.

Pregnancy is an obvious contraindication to this procedure. However, Honey, et al.[11] reported a case where embolization was done to treat bleeding from a cervical pregnancy while attempting to maintain a coexisting intrauterine pregnancy. The procedure was successful but after 10 days the fetus died. In a related case, Chen et al.[12] describes an unrecognized pregnancy that survived occlusion of the uterine vessels by laparoscopic coagulation. The pregnancy progressed four weeks before termination at the patient's request. Although this latter case suggests that pregnancy can survive the insult of uterine artery occlusion, it would be unjustifiable to use UAE in the face of an ongoing pregnancy with the possible rare exception of the first case above or similar situation.

It is illogical to use UAE for management of fibroids in the postmenopausal female since these women have reached the natural endpoint for this disease. The hypoestrogenic state of menopause reduces blood flow through the uterine arteries as well as individual myomas.[3] This change is responsible for the cessation of growth and symptoms normally seen when women achieve menopause. In fact, this effect that has led to the use of GnRH analogs and ultimately uterine artery occlusion as a means of treating this disease.

Patients with mild to moderate radiographic contrast allergies are normally managed with steroid administration whereas severe contrast allergy is viewed as a contraindication.[13]

Because contrast material must be cleared through the kidneys, renal impairment is viewed as a contraindication to UAE. A–V malformations involving the uterine arteries pose the risk of embolizing the venous system and ultimately to the lung. Fortunately, this malformation is rare and can be closed[14] from the venous side by the interventional radiologist allowing for subsequent UAE.

An undiagnosed pelvic mass is a contraindication for many reasons:

(1) It could represent active pelvic infection.
(2) UAE could delay, obscure, or prevent appropriate treatment of the mass.

The first major complication of UAE in the United States was caused by active pelvic infection.[15] This resulted in a life threatening flare up of the pelvic infection. A pelvic mass can represent a pregnancy, a pelvic kidney or an ovarian neoplasia. None of these is appropriately treated by UAE and, in the case of pelvic malignancy, unnecessary delay in treatment could result.

Table 13.5. Uterine artery embolization: future pregnancy concerns

• Compromise blood supply
• Compromise myometrial integrity
• Premature ovarian failure

The question, as to whether UAE should be performed in women who desire future pregnancy, is still unsettled. The most common concerns are listed in Table 13.5. Although multiple reports of successful pregnancy after occlusion of the uterine blood supply exist, they all suffer from inadequate numbers and appropriate controls.[10,16–19] As a consequence, if this procedure is to be offered to young women wishing future pregnancy, they must be fully informed about the potential risks.

Conclusion

As UAE has increased in use for management of symptomatic fibroids the need to define better and possibly narrow its indications has become apparent. With time and more data, we should be able to predict the response in specific situations and more accurately define those best suited for this treatment. It is quite possible that the applicability will broaden rather than narrow.

REFERENCES

1. Shlansky-Goldberg R (2000). Uterine artery embolization: historical and anatomic considerations. *Sem Interv Radiol* **17**: 223–36.
2. Ravina JH, Bouret JM, Fried D, et al. (1995). Value of preoperative embolization of uterine fibroma: report of a multicenter series of 31 cases. *Contracept Fertil Sex* **23**: 45–9.
3. Matta WHM, Stabile I, Shaw RW, et al. (1988). Doppler assessment of uterine blood flow in patients with fibroids receiving gonadotropin-releasing hormone agonist buserlin. *Fertil Steril* **49**: 1083.
4. Stoval TG, Muneyyirci-Delale O, Summitt RL, Jr & Scialli AR, et al. (1995). GnRH agonist and iron versus placebo and iron in the anemic patient before surgery for leiomyomas: a randomized controlled trial. *Obstet Gynecol* **86**: 65–71.

5. Hutchins FL, Worthington-Kirsch RL & Berkowitz RP (1999). Selective uterine artery embolization as primary treatment for symptomatic leiomyomata uteri: a review of 305 consecutive cases. *J Am Assoc Gynecol Laparosc* **6**(3): 279–84.

6. Ravina JH, Aymard A, Ciraru-Vigneron N, et al. (1998). Embolisation artérielle particulaire: un nouveau traitement des hémorragies des léiomyomes utérins. *Presse Med* **27**: 299–303.

7. Worthington-Kirsch R, personal communication March, 2002.

8. Hemingway AP (1991). Complications of embolotherapy. In *Current Practice of Interventional Radiology*, S. Kadir (ed.), pp. 104–8. BC Decker, Inc. Philadelphia.

9. Greenwood CH, Glickman MG, Schwartz PE, Morse SS & Denny DF (1987). Obstetric and nonmalignant gynecologic bleeding: treatment with angiographic embolization. *Radiology* **164**: 155–9.

10. Wilms G, Peene P & Baert AL (1990). Transcatheter arterial embolization in the management of gynecologic bleeding. *J Belge Radiol* **73**: 21–5.

11. Honey L, Leader A & Claman P (1999). Uterine artery embolization – a successful treatment to control bleeding from cervical pregnancy with simultaneous intrauterine gestation. *Hum Reprod* **14**: 553–5.

12. Chen YJ, Wang PH, Yuan CC, et al. (2002). Early pregnancy uninterrupted by laparoscopic bi-polar coagulation of uterine vessels. *J Am Assoc Gynecol Laparosc* **9**: 79–83.

13. Hutchins FL & Worthington-Kirsch R (2000). Embolotherapy for myoma induced menorrhagia. *Obstet Gynecol Clin N Am* **27**(2): 397–405.

14. Arrendondo-Soberon F, Loret de Mola JR, Shlansky-Goldberg R & Tureck RW (1997). Uterine arteriovenous malformation in a patient with recurrent pregnancy loss and a bicornuate uterus: a case report. *J Reprod Med* **42**: 239–43.

15. Goodwin SC, Vedantham S, McLucas B, et al. (1997). Uterine artery embolization for treatment of uterine fibroids: results of a pilot study. *J Vasc Interv Radiol* **8**: 517–26.

16. Stancato-Pasik A, Mitty HA, Richard HM III & Eshkar NS (1996). Obstetric embolotherapy: effect on menses and pregnancy. *Radiology* **201**(P): 179.

17. McIvor J & Cameron EW (1996). Pregnancy after uterine artery embolization to control hemorrhage from gestational trophoblastic tumor. *Br J Radiol* **69**: 624–9.

18. McLucas B, Goodwin S, Adler L, et al. (2001). Pregnancy following uterine fibroid embolization. *Int J Obstet Gynecol* **74**(1): 1–7.

19. Ravina JH, Vigneron NC, Aymard A, et al. (2000). Pregnancy after embolization of uterine myoma: report of 12 cases. *Fertil Steril* **73**(6): 1241–3.

14

Results of uterine artery embolization

Bruce McLucas

UCLA Medical Center, Los Angles, CA, USA

The first embolization for symptomatic myomata in Los Angeles was performed on November 24, 1994, at the University of California. The patients' bleeding following myomectomy was diminished using gelfoam delivered via arterial catheter. This began a collaboration between interventional radiologists and gynecologists for the treatment of symptomatic myomata using uterine artery embolization (UAE). During this study period, the technique of UAE has undergone some changes mainly due to the increasing experience of the interventional radiologists. Changes include the amount of devascularization, size of particles, and the introduction of new embolic materials.

Since the beginning of the procedure, our group has expanded to several interventional radiologists, and three types of facilities have been used to conduct the procedure. For the purpose of this review, we have evaluated whether the outcome of UAE is operator dependent or affected by the type and amount of particles used. We now have a five-year follow-up of women who have undergone the procedure. We have evaluated the long-term effects of embolization and the need for subsequent surgery. This chapter concentrates on analysis of results. We will briefly report our failures, and then reexamine them in Chapter 17.

Pre-embolization evaluation

Pre- and postmenopausal women are eligible if they have symptomatic uterine fibroid. We inform the potential patients about the lack of long-term follow up, and alternative treatment modalities. Screening of patients includes laboratory testing, such as coagulation profile and renal function. Contraindications to embolization are active infection, active bleeding, acute bleeding diasthesis, history of pelvic irradiation, life-threatening contrast allergy, poorly controlled diabetes, and abnormal kidney functions. All patients undergo pre-embolization imaging, either by ultrasound, or magnetic resonance, within three months of the procedure. In our institution, all patients are screened by laparoscopy and hysteroscopy prior to UAE. During hysteroscopy, biopsy of the myometrium is performed using the technique suggested by McCausland.[1]

Technique

The technique of embolization used by each operator varies little from the onset of the study to the present. Most patients underwent embolization under conscious sedation, and some under general anesthesia. First, local anesthesia is injected into the skin overlying the femoral artery on the right groin. The artery is punctured with either a one-sided or double-sided technique depending on the operator preference. A guide wire is inserted, and over that wire, a 5 French catheter is advanced. Operators have different preferences for catheter types, but all catheters have a memory with a bend at the tip. Under angiographic guidance, the patient's left iliac artery is entered, and then the hypogastric artery is followed into its anterior division. At this point

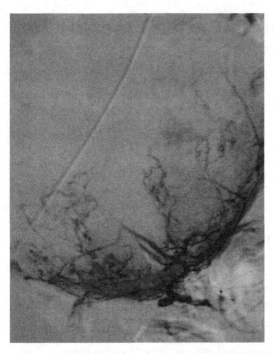

Figure 14.1. Right uterine artery supplying a myoma. Note the "open hand" pattern. (Courtesy of Louis Adler, MD.)

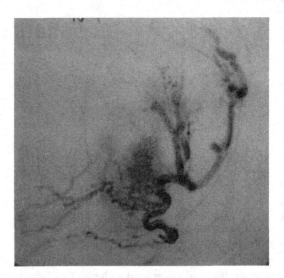

Figure 14.2. Deposit of contrast within myoma known as "blushing." This is nearing the endpoint of embolization. (Courtesy of Louis Adler, MD.)

some operators routinely insert a co-axial 3 French catheter through the outer catheter to identify and enter the uterine artery, while others proceed directly into the uterine artery with the original catheter. The uterine artery has an unmistakable medial course branching like an open hand around the myomata (Figure 14.1).

Embolization is done under fluoroscopic guidance. Using a "free-flow" technique, the operator injects small bursts of particles until the end point of embolization is reached. That end point has changed over the course of our series. Signs of relative stasis include a residual deposit of contrast stained particles known as "blushing" (Figure 14.2). Also, the rate of flow of injected particles slows as the distal branches become blocked. When reflux of injected particles occurs around the tip of the catheter, the operator knows that embolization is nearly completed. He or she will then inject cautiously, particles escape around the catheter tip putting the ovarian arteries at risk for ischemia.

Following embolization of the left artery, the right side is cannulated. In order to reach the right uterine artery, some physicians form a "Waldman loop" in the catheter, and then pull the looped catheter into the uterine artery. Others simply pull back on the catheter, and attempt to enter the right side directly. Once in place, the right artery is occluded.

From an interventional radiologist's point of view, the technique seems simple. There are numerous differences in approaches and considerable angiographic safety measures applied. This chapter is not intended to be a detailed guide, but an overview for practitioners.

Most patients receive pre-procedure antibiotics intravenously, usually Cefazolin. Before embolization of the right uterine artery, the patient is given Ketorolac 30 mg intramuscularly. Another 30 mg is given prior to discharge from the hospital. After embolization, pressure is applied to the femoral puncture for 10 minutes to prevent hematoma formation.

Embolization particles

Interventional radiologists have a wide range of temporary and permanent embolic agents. This depends

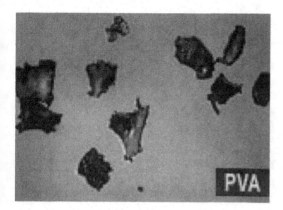

Figure 14.3. Polyvinyl alcohol particles (PVA). (Courtesy of Boston Scientific.)

on the goal of embolization and the organ they are embolizing. Permanent embolic agents include embolic particles and thrombogenic coils, a resin like material that moulds itself to the distal arterioles. Temporary embolization may be achieved with cut-up gelfoam cellulose sponges and injected into the uterine arteries. Although some centers have reported success using gelfoam,[2,3] this has not been the experience of others.[4] The duration of ischemic insult to the myoma that leads to permanent ischemia unresponsive to hormonal stimuli is unknown.

Most radiologists use permanent materials for UAE. Some have used coils to embolize vessels in gynecological and obstetrical conditions.[4] Coils prevent future access to the same artery. Because re-embolization is sometimes needed, we prefer to use embolic particles. Some physicians choose to "top off" with gelfoam pieces. Gelfoam would prevent the systolic force of the artery from packing the embolic load more distally into the uterine arteries.

The initial embolic agent is polyvinyl alcohol particles (PVA). These inert plastic beads resemble grains of sand, and are manufactured in various size ranges. They are not round (Figure 14.3) and can only be produced within certain tolerances. They are supplied in vials containing different sizes, such as 300–500 μ, or 900–1200 μ. Smaller particles exist, and are useful for neuroradiology work, but not for UAE.

From the beginning, we have been using 300 μ of PVA. Larger particles, 500, 700, or 900 μ-sized would

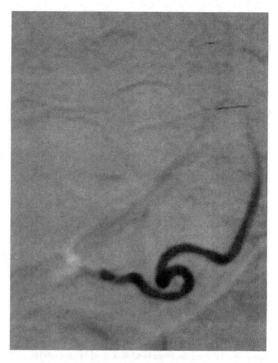

Figure 14.4. Complete occlusion of the uterine artery. (Courtesy of Louis Adler, MD.)

be injected on top of the smaller particles. The end point is occlusion of the artery, and reflux of the contrast back around the catheter (Figure 14.4). Over the years, two changes concerning particles emerged from ours and other centers. The first change was the amount of devascularization sought in UAE and the second change was the emergence of a new generation of embolic particle.

Post-embolization pain has been the most troublesome symptom of UAE. After the first year, we began to use larger particles, hoping to cause ischemia with minimal anoxia. Today, no physician uses a particle smaller than 500 μ of PVA and our group begins embolization with a 700 μ sized particle. A group in France suggests that 700 μ are the typical size of the arteriole of the uterine artery as it enters the myoma.[5] Thus, smaller particles will enter the myoma, but not necessarily block the artery carrying blood to the myoma.

Concerning the degree of devascularization, another important change occurred during our study

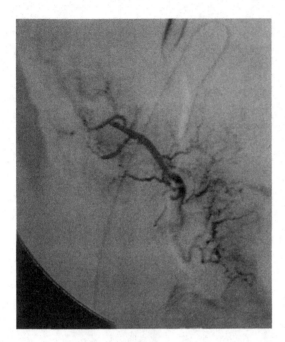

Figure 14.5. Subselective embolization of smaller arterioles, known as "Pruning the branches." (Courtesy of Louis Adler, MD.)

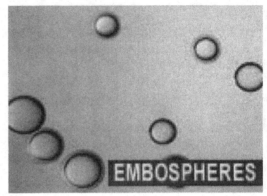

Figure 14.6. Embospheres. (Courtesy of Biosphere Medical, Inc.)

period. First, various centers reported the occurrence of premature menopause in a small percentage of patients.[6,7] The cause of this complication was thought to be reflux of particles beyond the tip of the catheter into the ovarian artery. In fact, several authors reported the discovery of particles in the ovarian arteries of hysterectomized women who had had UAE.[8]

To prevent reflux of the particles, less aggressive devascularization by slow injection of particles was done. Rather than complete occlusion, we intended to block the smaller arterioles, or "pruning the branches" of the uterine artery (Figure 14.5). We initiated this technique in 1998.

Until 1999, the embolic material was PVA. PVA had been used safely for all parts of the body for 20 years. PVA particles are not uniform in size, and it appears that they have a tendency to clump out of the catheter, thus do not travel as distal as the diameter of the particles would allow. Newer particles

for UAE – Embosphere – became available in 1999. Embospheres were uniform in shape (Figure 14.6) and resistant to the clumping phenomenon. We have used both types of particles, and both techniques (more vs. less aggressive devascularization). This has allowed us to examine whether particle type and size made a difference in shrinkage, as well as the difference in amount of devascularization. We have also calculated the "particle load" to occlude the uterine arteries used by each physician (vials of particles/liters of uterus embolized). We evaluated if individual changes in technique over the course of the study period made a difference in this calculation.

Setting

Initially, we performed UAE in a university hospital. Several cases were then successfully done in a community hospital. Today, we performed UAE on selected patients in an outpatient surgical center.

Follow up

Patients are seen within the first week after UAE. Repeat imaging and clinical evaluation are done at six weeks and again at six months after the procedure. We have observed shrinkage in several myomas,[9]

Table 14.1. Fibroid shrinkage over time

Time of imaging evaluation	n	Mean fibroid (cm)	% reduction	P-value
Pre-treatment	591	7.3		
6 weeks after UAE	400	6.2	15	0.0006
6 months after UAE	309	5.3	27	0.04
12 months after UAE	145	4.8	34	0.15
60 months after UAE	10	9.0	−19	0.1

UAE: uterine artery embolization.

beyond six months after the procedure. Patients are scheduled to undergo ultrasound imaging annually. This has allowed us to report our UAE results among a group of patients five years after their procedure. We became aware of adverse events including subsequent operations by periodic contact with patients.

We define failure as shrinkage less than two standard deviations from the average, persistence or worsening of symptoms, and subsequent hysterectomy. We will analyze our failure data in Chapter 17.

Fertility

After establishing that UAE was a safe procedure, we started offering it to women desiring fertility. Our study patients were those who desired to conceive but who were not infertile. Accordingly, we did not undertake infertility investigation.

Results

In this Chapter, we report our results from patients seen between November 1994 to November 2001. During this period, 5532 women enquired about UAE. We treated 595 (11%) pre- and postmenopausal women. Our patient population consisted of women with the mean age 43.1 years (range 21–67), gravidity 1.4 (range 0–10), and parity 0.7 (range 0–4). During pre-embolization evaluation, we excluded several patients. The reasons for exclusion are sarcoma, adenocarcinoma (endometrium), acute salpingitis, tubo-ovarian abscess, solid ovarian tumors, and atypical endometrial hyperplasia. The results of endoscopy examination prior to UAE are shown in Table 14.1. Special attention was given to pedunculated myomata. Due to the risks of necrosis of the subserous myoma and adhesion formation[10,11] these patients were offered laparoscopic myomectomy immediately after UAE. Women with pedunculated submucous myomata were warned about the possibility of prolapsing myoma per vagina.[12,13]

Five hundred and ninety-five women were referred for embolization. Of these 576 women (97%) underwent bilateral UAE successfully. Of the remaining 19 women, (3%) failed the initial embolization – 2 (11%) were unsuccessfully re-treated while 8 (42%) were subsequently embolized successfully. Nine patients refused a repeat embolization. One woman experienced an arterial tear requiring vascular surgery. There were no other procedural complications. We changed the extent of devascularization in 1999.

Immediate post-embolization period

Four hundred and thirty women (72%) had UAE in a hospital setting. Ten women underwent a combination of embolization and laparoscopic procedure. Of 420 women (71%) who underwent UAE only the average hospital stay was 24 hours and 173 women (29%) underwent UAE in the outpatient setting. Of these, 9 women (5%) were admitted overnight for observation; 164 women (95%) who did not require extended observation, had an average stay of less than eight hours. There is no difference in the average length of stay between the hospital setting and the outpatient setting. This 95% success rate encourages us to recommend UAE as an outpatient procedure.

Among the outpatient population, 9 (5%) women were readmitted. Two women were readmitted for pain control, and four for evaluation of post-embolization fever. Most readmissions for fever occurred in the first year of our study. Subsequently, we evaluated our patients as an outpatient basis. Patients were told to stay off work and perform light activity for one week. One patient who went jogging the day after UAE developed a groin hematoma.

Many authors have reported postembolization pain. Intravenous or intramuscular narcotics can manage it. Similar pain has been reported as a result of embolization performed for other organs of the body.[14,15,16] The pain was thought to be ischemic in type. This is similar to the pain due to decreased oxygenation of the myocardium in patients with myocardial ischemia. Together with temperature elevation, and possible nausea, the condition is referred to as "post embolization syndrome."[17,18] Post-embolization pain is most intense immediately after UAE, and becomes less severe with the passage of hours on the day of the procedure. The pain is not related to the size of the uterus, or of the amount of particles administered.

Passage of submucous myomata

Of the 107 patients who were found to have pedunculated submucous myomata at the time of pre embolization hysteroscopy, 17 (16%) reported symptoms of passing necrotic myomata. Symptoms included green and foul smelling discharge, crampy pain, and return of menorrhagia. We performed a vaginal myomectomy to complete the passage of the myomata. Of note, laparoscopy performed concomitantly with the vaginal myomectomy showed no evidence of salpingitis.

Shrinkage

We used two measurements, the largest diameter of the dominant myoma, and the total uterine volume

(TUV). TUV was calculated using the volume of a prolate ellipse (length × width × depth × 0.52). Most of our patients had imaging follow-ups, six weeks and six months after UAE, some had a longer follow up.

The mean fibroid size before UAE was 7.3 cm and six months after was 5.3 cm. This exhibits a shrinkage of 27% ($P = 0.001$). The mean fibroid size at six weeks was 6.2 cm (15% shrinkage from baseline), 5.3 cm (27% shrinkage from baseline) at six months, and 4.8 cm (34% shrinkage from baseline) at 12 months. The results of this analysis are shown in Table 14.1. The mean difference between fibroid size at baseline and at different timepoints was statistically significant (repeated measure ANOVA, $P = 0.00001$). These results show that not only is the overall shrinkage of the fibroid significant, but the comparisons between individual time periods also exhibit significant shrinkage.

We also evaluated the mean shrinkage in TUV. The mean TUV at baseline and at six months was 688.3 cm and 348.2 cm, respectively. This exhibits a shrinkage of 49% ($P = 0.001$). The mean TUV at six weeks was 475.6 cm (31% shrinkage from baseline), 348.2 cm (49%) at six months, 342 (50%) at 12 months, and 184.5 cm (73%) at five years. We found significant shrinkage ($P = 0.00001$) between time periods (Table 14.2 and Figure 14.7). No patients experienced regrowth of myomata or growth of new myomas.

In patients with adenomyosis diagnosed at the time of hysteroscopy, the average shrinkage of the TUV and the uterine fibroid was 42.3% and 28.0% at six months, and 43.3% and 28.3% among those without adenomyosis respectively. As adenomyosis is a factor associated with UAE failure, it is expected that with larger samples the difference in shrinkage between patients with and without adenomyosis will become statistically significant. Given the association between deep adenomyosis on biopsy and hysterectomy, we estimated that the success rate of UAE among women with adenomyosis would be 50% compared to 90% among those without adenomyosis.

We evaluated several parameters that might affect the shrinkage including the operator, particle load, particle type, and particle size (Table 14.3). Our results showed that this parameter does not

Table 14.2. Total uterine volume (TUV) shrinkage over time

Time of imaging evaluation	n	Mean TUV (ml)	% reduction	P-value
Pretreatment	586	688.3		
6 weeks after UAE	395	475.6	31	0.00001
6 months after UAE	309	348.2	49	0.0001
12 months after UAE	143	342.0	50	0.8
60 months after UAE	10	184.5	73	0.01

UAE: uterine artery embolization.

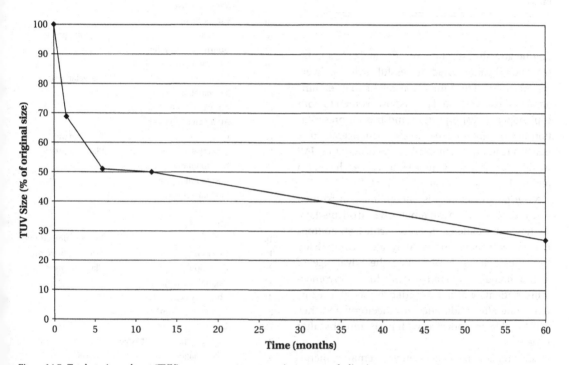

Figure 14.7. Total uterine volume (TUV) measurements post-uterine artery embolization.

influence the TUV or the fibroid shrinkage. The place of the procedure either private institution or university hospital did not alter the outcomes.

Fertility

Traditional wisdom states that myomata cause prematurity and pregnancy loss,[19,20,21] even though some authors claim better results of in vitro fertilization when myomata are not present.[22] We did not attempt to analyze our patient population for other risk factors for fertility. We simply asked the patients if they wished to maintain their fertility – 195 women responded positively. We drew an arbitrary line at age 40 years, believing that, beyond that age, multiple other factors play important roles in conception. In our population, 86 women under 40 desired fertility – 26 patients have conceived[23] (Table 14.4). Several features are striking about this group. No patient experienced uterine rupture either during pregnancy or labor. There were no reports of either intra

Table 14.3. Total uterine volume (TUV) shrinkage by operator, particle load, particle type and particle size

Shrinkage factor	P-value	
	TUV	Fibroid
Operator	0.4	0.3
Particle load	0.2	0.6
Particle type	0.4	0.2
Particle size	0.7	0.1

Table 14.4. Patients who conceived following uterine artery embolization

Patient	Delivery type	C-section indications
1	Lost to follow up[a]	
2	Lost to follow up[a]	
3	C-section	Placenta previa
4	C-section	Cephalopelvic disproportion
5	C-section	Repeat C-section
5	Vaginal delivery	
6	Currently pregnant	
6	C-section	Placenta previa
7	Abortion (<20 weeks)	
8	Vaginal delivery	
9	C-section	Pre-eclampsia
10	Vaginal delivery	
11	Abortion (<20 weeks)	
12	Abortion (<20 weeks)	
12	C-section	Placenta previa
13	C-section	Placenta previa
14	Lost to follow up[a]	
15	Lost to follow up[a]	
16	Vaginal delivery	
17	Miscarriage	
17	Miscarriage	
18	C-section	Prior myomectomy
19	C-section	Prior myomectomy
20	C-section	Placenta previa
20	Vaginal delivery	
21	Abortion (<20 weeks)	
22	Lost to follow up[a]	
23	Lost to follow up[a]	
24	Currently pregnant (twins)	
25	Miscarriage	15 weeks
26	Lost to follow up[a]	

[a]Patients were followed post uterine artery embolization and confirmed pregnant. Obstetric care provided by another physician
C-section: Cesarean section

uterine growth restriction, or of fetal distress in labor. Several patients had successful vaginal deliveries. We noted that diminution rather than elimination of myomata would predispose women to both cephalopelvic disproportion and breech presentation, leading to cesarean deliveries. Our overall pregnancy rate in women under 40 years of age after UAE was 30.2% (26 of 86 patients). Other centers have also reported successful pregnancy after UAE.[24]

More pregnancy loss is encountered in women with uterus of $\geq$20 cm in diameter. Based on this data, we now offer patients desiring fertility an abdominal myomectomy immediately after UAE. Using this approach we have gained the advantage of a near bloodless operative field during myomectomy. Patients will not experience the 30% recurrence rate after traditional myomectomy and they will be able to conceive within six months after surgery.

Some patients have experienced premature menopause after UAE. In our population, 47 (7.9%) women experienced a rise in serum follicle stimulating hormone (FSH) to menopausal levels within six months of their procedure. None of them was younger than 40 years, while 30 patients were older than 45 years. Among women >45 years with increasing serum FSH levels, the levels returned to normal in five women and they continued to menstruate. Among 17 women between the ages of 40 and 45 years, the FSH levels returned to normal within 12 months in eight, remained elevated in five women, and four women were lost to follow-up. In our patient population, the risks of premature menopause is 0.8% (5 of 595). This complication is due to overzealous injection of particles. In one patient undergoing hysterectomy and unilateral salpingo-oophorectomy immediately after UAE, embolic particles were found in the ovarian artery (Figure 14.8).

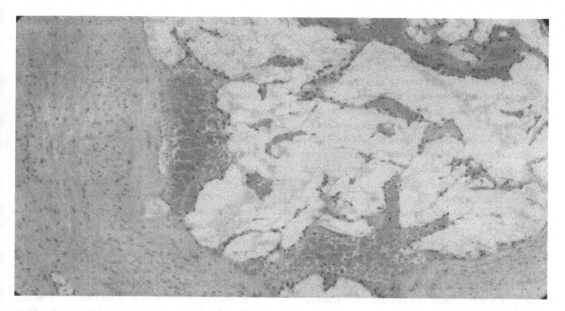

Figure 14.8. Embolic particles noted in ovarian artery following hysterectomy.

Other centers have reported higher rates of premature ovarian failure.[25] Recent changes in the technique throughout the world have reduced this complication. The amount of radiation exposure to the ovaries in 50 of our patients was 14 rads,[10] not a worrisome level.

Comments

To date, we have followed 40 patients who underwent UAE more than five years ago. The initial shrinkage has continued or held steady in all patients. Thirty-nine patients reported continued symptom relief. One patient has undergone a hysterectomy after the five-year period but was diagnosed with adenomyosis at the time of initial hysteroscopy. UAE appears to permanently shrink the myomata, and prevent new myomata from forming. After five years, shrinkage of both TUV and fibroid size continued, although not as fast as the shrinkage in the first year after UAE. This long-term data gives further evidence of the permanence of UAE.

Other centers with long-term data reported similar efficacy after five years.[26] Based on estimates of suppliers of embolic materials, the number of cases of UAE performed worldwide is thought to be approaching 50 000. We anticipate a number of reports to be forthcoming to bolster our findings.

REFERENCES

1. McCausland AM (1992). Hysteroscopic myometrial biopsy: its use in diagnosing adenomyosis and its clinical application. *Am J Obstet Gynecol* **166**: 1619–28.
2. Katsumori T, Nakajima K, Mihara T & Tokuhiro M (2002). Uterine artery embolization using gelatin sponge particles alone for symptomatic uterine fibroids: midterm results. *Am J Roentgenol* **178**(1): 135–9.
3. Stancato-Pasik A, Katz R, Mitty HA, Cooper J, Ahn J, Braffman B, Carano K & Brodman M (1999). Uterine artery embolisation of myomas: preliminary results of gelatin sponge pledgets as the embolic agent. *Min Invas Ther & Allied Technol* **8**(6): 393–6.
4. Abbas F, Currie J, Mitchell S, Osterman F, Rosenshein N & Horowitz I (1994). Selective vascular embolization in benign gynecologic conditions. *J Reprod Med* **39**: 4926.
5. Pelage JP, Ferrand J, Wassef M, et al. (2001). Combined embolization and myomectomy for symptomatic uterine fibroids. *Cardi Vasc Interv Radiol* **24**: 142 (Abstract.)

6. Bradley EA, Reidy JF, Forman RG, Jarosz J & Braude PR (1998). Transcatheter uterine artery embolisation to treat large uterine fibroids. *Br J Obstet Gynaecol* **105**: 235–40.

7. Klein A & Schwartz ML (2001). Uterine artery embolization for the treatment of uterine fibroids: an outpatient procedure. *Am J Obstet Gynecol* **184**(7): 1556–60.

8. Walker W, Green A & Sutton C (1999). Bilateral uterine artery embolisation for myomata: results, complications and failures. *Min Invas Ther & Allied Technol* **8**(6): 449–54.

9. McLucas B, Adler L & Perrella R (2001). Uterine fibroid embolization: nonsurgical treatment for symptomatic fibroids. *J Am Coll Surg* **192**(1): 95–105.

10. Godfrey CD & Zbella EA (2001). Uterine necrosis after uterine artery embolization for leiomyoma. *Obstet Gynecol* **98**(5, Pt 2): 950–2.

11. McLucas B, Goodwin S & Vedantham S (1996). Embolic therapy for myomata. *Min Invas Ther Allied Technol* **5**: 336–8.

12. Abbara S, Spies JB, Scialli AR, Jha RC, Lage JM & Nikolic B (1999). Transcervical expulsion of a fibroid as a result of uterine artery embolization for leiomyomata. *J Vasc Interv Radiol* **10**: 409–11.

13. Berkowitz RP, Hutchins FL & Worthington-Kirsch RL (1999). Vaginal expulsion of submucosal fibroids after uterine artery embolization. *J Reprod Med* **44**: 373–6.

14. Watanabe S, Minami A, Nishioka M, Ohkawa M & Koui F et al. (1997). Left brachial approach for transcatheter embolization therapy in patients with hepatocelluar carcinoma. *Dig Dis Sci* **42**: 47–58.

15. Slomka M & Radwan P (1992). The evaluation of clinical results of hepatic artery embolization. *Mater Med Pol* **24**: 193–5.

16. Chung JW, Park JH, Han JK, et al. (1996). Hepatic tumors: predisposing factors for complications of transcatheter oily chemoembolization. *Radiology* **198**: 33–40.

17. McLucas B & Rappoport AS (1999). Transcatheter uterine fibroid embolisation for uterine fibroids using a mobile fluoroscopy unit in an out-patient surgical center. *Min Invas Ther & Allied Technol* **8**(6): 433–6.

18. Worthington-Kirsch RL, Popky GL & Hutchins FL (1998). Uterine arterial embolization for the management of leiomyomas: quality-of-life assessment and clinical response. *Radiology* **208**: 625–9.

19. Benson CB, Chow JS, Chang-Lee W, Hill JA, III & Doubilet PM (2001). Outcome of pregnancies in women with uterine leiomyomas identified by sonography in the first trimester. *J Clin Ultrasound* **29**(5): 261–4.

20. Salvador E, Bienstock J, Blakemore KJ & Pressman E (2002). Leiomyomata uteri, genetic amniocentesis, and the risk of second-trimester spontaneous abortion. *Am J Obstet Gynecol* **186**(5, Pt 1): 913–15.

21. Vergani P, Ghidini A, Strobelt N, Roncaglia N, Locatelli A, Lapinski RH & Mangioni C (1994). Do uterine leiomyomas influence pregnancy outcome? *Am J Perinatol* **11**(5): 356–8.

22. Hart R, Khalaf Y, Yeong CT, Seed P, Taylor A & Braude P (2001). A prospective controlled study of the effect of intramural uterine fibroids on the outcome of assisted conception. *Hum Reprod* **16**(11): 2411–17.

23. McLucas B, Goodwin S, Adler L, Rappaport A, Reed R & Perrella R (2001). Pregnancy following uterine fibroid embolization. *Int J Gynaecol Obstet* **74**: 1–7.

24. Ravina JH, Vigneron NC, Aymard A, et al. (2000). Pregnancy after embolization of uterine myoma: a report of 12 cases. *Fertil Steril* **73**(6): 1241–3.

25. Stinger NH, Grant T, Park J & Oldham L (2000). Ovarian failure after uterine artery embolization for treatment of myomas. *J Am Assoc Gynecol Laparosc* **7**(3): 395–400.

26. Ravina JH, Ciraru-Vigneron N, Aymard A, Ferrand J & Merland JJ (1999). Uterine artery embolisation for fibroid diseases: results of a 6 year study. *Min Invas Ther & Allied Technol* **8**(6): 441–7.

15

Side effects and complications of embolization

George A. Vilos

The University of Western Ontario, Ontario, Canada

Introduction

Uterine artery embolization (UAE) has been introduced as a treatment option of uterine leiomyomas because it preserves the uterus and may avoid some of the risks associated with hysterectomy or myomectomy.[1] The therapy is performed in the medical imaging (or radiology) department by interventional radiologists. Although it is considered minimally invasive therapy it does carry its own inherent side effects and potential complications. Side effects may be unavoidable and occur as the result or a consequence of the intended treatment while complications are abnormal conditions that occur during or following the treatment.

The side effects and complications of UAE can be classified as intra-operative and postoperative. Although minor side effects are experienced by virtually all patients undergoing the embolization treatment, major complications are rare, experienced by less than 1% of patients.[2–7] Although this complication rate is much lower than the rates associated with hysterectomy and myomectomy some complications can be potentially serious and they should be fully disclosed to the patients.

It should be noted that since UAE is a relatively new procedure (less than 10 years old), some complications may be new and the therapists should maintain a high index of suspicion and be alert for unusual and unconventional signs and symptoms to avoid misdiagnosis of serious conditions.

Peri-operative risks and complications

Puncture site complications

Infection, bleeding, and hematoma formation at the groin puncture site have been reported to occur at a frequency of less than 1%.[2–7] Bleeding is usually managed by applying pressure while in the recovery room patients are instructed to keep their legs straight for four to six hours, and to refrain from coughing. After six to eight hours the patients are discharged or transferred to the ward and they may be up and about.

Allergic/anaphylactic reactions

Allergies to the iodinated contrast dye and to medications given for sedation and analgesia can occur and they range from mild to life threatening events. Allergic reactions are encountered by about 1% of patients, with severe reactions much rarer.[2]

Incomplete UAE catheterization

Successful bilateral UAE has been reported in 92% to 98% of patients.[2–9] From the published reports and our own experience involving >500 patients, catheterization of the uterine arteries is successful bilaterally in approximately 97% of cases, unilaterally in 2–3% and unsuccessful in 0.5–1% of cases. Factors associated with inability to catheterize the uterine arteries include anatomic variations, small tortuous arteries, arterial spasm, intimal dissection, and operator experience and expertise.

Misembolization

Fluoroscopically the ovarian arteries as they approach the ovary and the uterine arteries are easily recognized due to their distinct corkscrew shape.[2] However, due to anatomical variations, aberrant arteries or inadequate experience and expertise, misembolization may occur. Misembolization refers to a situation when polyvinyl alcohol (PVA) particles go to other organs unintentionally. Although this can be a serious problem it is extremely rare due to the extent of collateralization in the pelvic circulation. Potential non-target embolization can result in ovarian dysfunction and adjacent organ ischemia or even necrosis.[2] Indeed, following UAE for the treatment of fibroids, one case of bladder and bilateral distal ureteral necrosis has been encountered in Canada. To minimize the risk for misembolization, arteriography must be performed to ensure safe catheter position and to confirm that no vascular anomalies or aberrant vessels are present.[2–9] The presence of a significant arteriovenous shunting may send PVA particles into the venous system of the circulation with potential consequences to the pulmonary system.

Radiation exposure

The average time required to perform bilateral UAE has been reported to be approximately one hour.[2–9] However, the median fluoroscopy time required to complete the procedure is 15–30 minutes and this radiation exposure is comparable to that required to complete some diagnostic procedures such as barium enema.

Post-procedure side effects and complications

Acute post-embolization pain

There are two elements of pain associated with UAE. The first is the angiography and catheterization of the appropriate artery and the second, and by far the most painful, is the ischemia of the uterus and myomas following the embolization. As a rule, selective angiography in adults can be completed with local anesthesia alone, or local anesthesia plus conscious sedation.

Following UAE almost all patients experience some degree of acute or early labor-like crampy pain requiring specific management protocols and monitoring.[2] No correlation has been established between uterine size, myoma number or size, duration of procedure, quantity of PVA particles used, or clinical outcome of the treatment.[2] Embolization of the uterine arteries causes nonspecific ischemia to the uterus and the uterine fibroids. The immediate abdominal pain and cramps are most likely related to ischemia of both the uterus and its fibroids. The uterus has a very rich anastomotic blood supply from the uterine and ovarian arteries allowing reperfusion after the initial insult of ischemia while most myomas have a less vascular anastomotic network than the adjacent myometrium leading to degeneration and necrosis. As a rule the myometrium survives the acute ischemic episode undamaged while the myomas undergo hyaline degeneration and necrosis.[2] A second component to the early pain may be a generalized inflammatory reaction. The initial pain is self-limiting and usually resolves within two days to two weeks. Protocols for pain management include pre-emptive analgesia consisting of preoperative administration of non-steroidal anti-inflammatory drugs (NSAIDS) followed by postoperative NSAIDS in conjunction with patient controlled analgesia (PCA) for administration of morphine and other narcotics. The insertion of epidural catheters prior to the embolization, and continue for the next 24–48 hours, has also been practiced in some centers. Hospitalization may require a 2–4 day extension strictly for pain control, however, in our study the vast majority of patients were discharged the morning following embolization.

Post-embolization syndrome

As noted above, most patients experience some degree of abdominal and/or pelvic pain following UAE. However, up to 40% of patients experience a variety of signs and symptoms including diffuse abdominal pain, generalized malaise, anorexia, nausea, vomiting, low-grade fever, and leukocytosis.[3-7] This has been referred to as the post-UAE syndrome and it is experienced by approximately one-third of the patients within the first 48 hours.[2-10] Up to 15% of patients require hospitalization longer than 24 hours for this syndrome. Low grade fever is experienced by approximately one-third of patients[4] while white blood cell count (WBC) upwards of 30×10^9/l may occur.[10] The syndrome is self-limiting and usually resolves within 48 hours with conservative and supportive therapy consisting of intravenous fluids and adequate pain control including NSAIDS. Antibiotics for the low grade fever and leukocytosis are usually not required unless there is clear evidence of septicemia.

The pathogenesis of leukocytosis and fever is probably related to the release of endogenous cytokines such as interleukin-1, interleukin-6, tumor necrosis factor, and interferon from acutely ischemic and necrosing fibroids.[11-12]

Infection

In general, postoperative febrile morbidity is defined as two temperature elevations greater than 38 °C, taken six hours apart, excluding the first 24 hours. The incidence of febrile morbidity and sepsis following embolization has been reported to be between 1.0% and 1.8%.[5,13-14] The infections have been shown to be pyometra with endomyometritis, bilateral chronic salpingitis, tubo-ovarian abscess, and infected myomas. Concomitant or pre-existing urinary tract infections appear to be co-morbidity factors. The most frequent pathogen isolated is *Escherischia coli* although other enterococcal bacteria have been implicated in urosepsis and endomyometritis.

Although infections following embolotherapy are rare, they can have serious consequences and require prolonged hospitalization, intensive therapy and even a hysterectomy and bilateral salpingo-oophorectomy. Some cases do respond to antibiotic therapy and do not require hysterectomy. These patients are usually passing necrotic submucous

fibroids. On the other hand, fulminant infections may lead to extreme consequences including death. Indeed one patient died 22 days following embolization from *E. coli* urosepsis despite an abdominal hysterectomy performed seven days after embolization and intensive therapy.[15]

Because of the potential serious consequences of infection, prophylactic intravenous or intra-arterial antibiotics have been advocated by some therapists. So far there are no randomized clinical trials to support or refute the benefits of prophylactic antibiotics. Opinions are mixed among the therapists and their use is based on personal bias, preference, and experience. Prophylactic antibiotics should be reserved for patients at higher risk of infection according to established guidelines.[16]

Persistent or chronic pain

In 5–10% of patients the pain persists over two weeks.[6-7] When the pain persists after two months of embolization and it is severe enough to require analgesic medication and interferes with the patient's normal functions and activities, a hysterectomy may be indicated. Underlying causes for persistent pain are unclear but nonspecific pre-existing factors such as prior laparotomy for myomectomy or history of inflammatory bowel disease with intestinal obstruction and adhesions have been implicated. Persistent pain, in the absence of infection, does not resolve spontaneously and as a rule may require surgical intervention. Hysterectomy for post-embolization pain has been reported in up to 2% of women.[9,17] One of our patients continued to experience severe post-UAE pain and at two months she expelled through the cervix a $6.5 \times 3.5 \times 2.0$ cm necrotic myoma. However, the pain persisted and following hysterectomy at four months post-embolization the uterus weighed 140 g and the histology demonstrated an extensively infracted endomyometrium with foreign body emboli present.

Ovarian dysfunction

Transient and permanent menopausal symptoms indicative of ovarian failure have been reported by up to 5% of women after UAE.[5,18-21] One study compared pre-embolization serum levels of follicle stimulating hormone (FSH) from 66 women, with 29 samples available at three months and 13 samples available at six months following embolization. Although the serum FSH level increased more than one standard deviation in 4 (6%) of 66 women three months after the procedure no statistical difference was found from the base line mean of 8.0 IU/l compared with the measurements at three and six months.[7]

Underlying factors leading to ovarian dysfunction are unknown. The evidence to date indicates that older patients, more than 45 years of age, are more likely to experience post-embolization ovarian dysfunction. Radiation exposure to the ovaries has been theorized to be one potential mechanism. However, a correlation between fluoroscopy exposure and frequency of ovarian dysfunction has not been established. One study involving 23 patients reported that the average radiation to the ovaries during embolization was estimated to be 30–100 times higher than that during routine diagnostic X-rays.[19] Such moderate radiation exposure during embolotherapy may cause chromosomal breaks in the ova, compromise ovarian reserve and adversely effect subsequent fertility and pregnancy outcomes.

The most likely mechanism leading to ovarian dysfunction seems to be ovarian misembolization via the utero-ovarian anastomotic vasculature.[5–6] Such anastomotic arteries have been demonstrated in up to 17% of cases during selective uterine artery angiography.[2] Ovarian failure is thought to occur more frequently when small PVA (150–250 μm) particles are used[10] and indeed such particles have been identified in ovarian vessels following hysterectomy in one patient after embolization of the uterine arteries.[2]

The consequences of premature ovarian failure have not been clearly elucidated. When preservation of fertility is still desired ovarian failure is of greater consequence while induction of an early menopause may be a welcome event by women suffering from abnormal uterine bleeding. In addition, the issue of hormone replacement therapy (HRT) post-UAE remains unknown. It has been demonstrated that leiomyomas do not increase in size after administration of post-menopausal HRT.[22] Based on the above evidence it stands to reason that leiomyomas will be even less likely to increase after embolotherapy in women requiring HRT. However, data to support this hypothesis have not been published.

Menstrual dysfunction

Abnormal uterine bleeding together with pelvic or abdominal pain has been reported to be the main indication for UAE in approximately two-thirds of patients. The available evidence indicates that there is improvement in menstrual bleeding in up to 89% of women following UAE.[2] The menstrual improvement is highly age dependent, being the highest after the age of 50 years. Transient and permanent amenorrhea has been reported to be approximately 15%[5,7,23–24] and 3%[7,23] of women, respectively. Amenorrhea after embolotherapy is also highly age dependent. In our own studies, the rate increased gradually to reach approximately 10% by the age of 50 years and jumped to over 40% after the age of 50. Permanent amenorrhea is a major complication in women desiring fertility but it might be perceived as a successful treatment outcome in women with abnormal uterine bleeding whose desire to preserve their uterus and fertility is no longer an issue. To put this into perspective in our own study involving over 500 cases, 50% of women undergoing UAE were nulliparous and 30% wished to retain their fertility.

Abnormal uterine bleeding did not improve in a number of patients, ranging from 4% to 21%.[5,7,23–24] In addition a small percentage of women reported no significant change or worsening of menstrual bleeding including persistent vaginal serosanguinous discharge after UAE.[3] In these women hysteroscopic endometrial ablation and removal of necrotic myomas and evacuation of pus or even hysterectomies have been carried out.

Transcervical myoma expulsion

Following UAE spontaneous expulsion of myomas through the cervix has been reported to occur in approximately 5–7% of patients with one study reporting up to 18%.[25] In women with submucous myomas confirmed by hysteroscopy, 60% passed myomas vaginally.[26]

It has been observed that submucous myoma expulsion seems to occur more frequently in women who have received gonadotropin-releasing hormone (GnRH) analogs. The underlying mechanism appears to be uterine shrinkage forcing intramural myomas into the uterine cavity from where they can be expelled spontaneously by uterine contractions. We have experienced one case where a singular 8 cm submucous myoma was expelled in several necrotic pieces with complete restoration of the uterus and uterine cavity.

Uterine wall integrity

The physical characteristics, integrity, and the histopathologic features of the uterine wall after UAE remain unknown. Following UAE, devascularized and shrunken fibroids that were easily detachable from their cradle in the myometrium leaving deep myometrial defects have been seen during hysteroscopic examination. Uterine wall defects,[27] uterine fistula[28] and one case of diffuse uterine necrosis[29] following UAE have been reported.

For these reasons, in patients contemplating pregnancy the integrity and features of the uterine wall and cavity should be assessed by imaging and combined laparoscopy and hysteroscopy prior to undertaking pregnancy. The relationship of myomas to reproductive outcomes is not well characterized. Existing literatures suggests that myomas are the cause of infertility in a relatively small percentage of patients.[30] Independent association between leiomyomas and abruptio placenta, first trimester bleeding, breech presentation, and cesarean section rates have been observed.[31] However, whether embolization of the uterine artery enhances or compromises fertility and pregnancy outcomes remains unknown. Fertility may be affected by the size and location of the myomas, endometrial and myometrial perfusion as well as ovarian function.[29] Pregnancy and delivery rates do not appear to be compromised when intramural myomas smaller than 7 cm are present as long as there is no encroachment in the endometrial cavity.[32,33] Anecdotal normal pregnancies and deliveries following UAE for acute post-partum hemorrhage[34] and for treatment of myomas have been reported.[35]

Embolization in women with pelvic malignancies

There is no reason to believe that embolization of the uterine arteries initiates or promotes malignant changes in any of the pelvic organs. However, since the diagnosis of leiomyosarcoma is usually made after a hysterectomy or myomectomy the concern has been raised that embolotherapy might miss or delay the diagnosis of leiomyosarcomas and other uterine cancers. Patients requiring UAE usually present with a pelvic mass and abnormal uterine bleeding with or without pelvic pain. All these signs and symptoms also occur with leiomyosarcomas and in association with other neoplastic tumors within the pelvis. The incidence of leiomyosarcomas in women between the ages of 40 and 60 years, was found to be 1% (8 of 817) of women with presumed leiomyomas producing symptoms that necessitated hysterectomy.[36] In our own experience the average age of women undergoing embolization has been 43 years of age with a range of 19 to 56. It is imperative then that all necessary steps and diagnostic tests be taken to avoid misdiagnosis and inadvertent embolization of malignant lesions of the genital tract. Although ovarian lesions might be distinguished from leiomyomas by imaging, routine ultrasonography (including color Doppler) has not been found to be particularly reliable while magnetic resonance imaging (MRI) has demonstrated some usefulness in distinguishing benign versus malignant smooth muscle tumors. Ill-defined margins of uterine smooth muscle tumors on MRI is one sign suggestive of malignancy.[37] In general, cervical and endometrial pre- and malignant lesions can be detected by routine cytology and endometrial sampling. These tests should be performed according to established guidelines routinely in patients when clinically indicated and technically feasible prior to undergoing UAE. Indeed we have inadvertently performed embolization of the uterine arteries in one patient who subsequently was found to have an endometrial adenocarcinoma and in two patients with leiomyosarcomas.

Preliminary studies assessing the efficacy of percutaneous needle biopsy to establish the diagnosis of leiomyosarcoma have been reported.[38] However, the practice has not been accepted widely and indeed leiomyosarcomas have been embolized inadvertently.[39] Leiomyosarcomas tend to be present as a singular large uterine mass or to be confined to the largest of the multiple uterine masses. However, there are no reliable clinical characteristics to identify a leiomyosarcoma as opposed to a benign leiomyoma other than an accelerated rate of increase in size. Continued increase in size following UAE has been put forth as a sign suggesting possible malignancy.

Myomectomy

Following UAE, myomectomy is uncommonly performed in women who are still symptomatic and who require maintaining their fertility or wishing to retain their uterus. The indications include persistent symptoms of bleeding or those related to bulk effects such as pressure to the adjacent organs from inadequate myoma shrinkage. Although the need for a myomectomy may be perceived as a treatment failure by some patients, it is usually considered a successful treatment outcome by surgeons, since the myomectomy and reconstruction of the uterus is easier to perform in a nearly bloodless field. This is particularly true when a singular or a small number of myomas are encountered.

Hysterectomy

The ultimate failure of UAE is the need for subsequent hysterectomy regardless of the indication. Hysterectomies performed within three months of embolization are usually due to complications while those performed after six months of embolization are due to treatment failures. The rate of hysterectomy within six months of embolization has been reported to be within 1–2% and the indications include infection, persistent bleeding, persistent pain, fibroid prolapse, and uterine malignancy.[3,5,13,38]

The underlying factors leading to uterine artery embolization failure may be due to technical failures and under-embolization, misdiagnosis, and alternative blood supply to the myomas. Under-embolization may result in insufficient disruption of the vascular blood supply to the uterus and repeat angiography and re-embolization might be considered in these patients.

Adenomyosis may be difficult to distinguish from a fibroid mass and may coexist in 20–40% of patients presenting with pelvic pain and/or a pelvic mass.[40–41] Adenomyosis with or without endometrial polyps and co-existing endometriosis or other nongynecological pathologies can be an additional underlying factor for uterine artery embolization failure. Therefore patients presenting with chronic pelvic pain and excessive uterine bleeding with an enlarged uterus and no clear evidence of fibroids may not be ideal candidates for UAE.

Alternative blood supply or minimal blood supply in hypovascular or partially calcified fibroids may be other reasons when there is inadequate reduction of myomas following UAE.[42] It has been reported that for up to 4% of patients the fibroids may be at least partly supplied by the ovarian arteries.[2]

Mortality

No fatality has been reported in the United States or Canada following UAE. In Europe it is estimated that 2000 procedures have been performed and two deaths have been associated with UAE. In the United Kingdom the one fatality was associated with septicemia[15] while in Italy the one death was attributed to pulmonary embolism from a clot in the pelvic veins following embolization.[2] Thromboembolism is the leading cause of mortality and morbidity among hospitalized patients.[43] Deep vein thrombosis in patients with large uterine myomata has been described.[44] Significant characteristics of patients with thromboembolism include malignancy, prior history of deep vein thrombosis, anesthesia >5 hours, prior pelvic radiation, venous stasis and venous varicosities, and age >45 years.[43] Prophylaxis against thromboembolism includes graduated pneumatic or stockings compression, low-dose standard heparin or low molecular weight heparin.[43] However, the cost-effectiveness of prophylaxis in women undergoing UAE has not been evaluated. Furthermore anticoagulation could reduce the efficacy of embolotherapy. It is estimated that to the end of 2001 up to 12 000 embolizations have been performed in the United States and Canada. The combined mortality then would be approximately 2 per 14 000 procedures or 0.14 per 1000. To put this into perspective the mortality associated with hysterectomy and myomectomy in women of similar ages has been estimated to be 0.3 and 0.6 per 1000,[45] respectively.

Summary

UAE is an effective and durable alternative to hysterectomy in women with uterine fibroids. It has been found to significantly reduce menorrhagia, dysmenorrhea, and fibroid bulk-related effects in approximately 90% of women.[2] Although there is a reduction of 45% and 55% in total uterine and myoma volume, respectively within six months following embolization, long-term data are lacking.[2] The follow-up of these patients is of short duration, in the majority of cases less than five years, and the long-term effects and complications associated with embolization have not yet been established. Since scientific data are limited, the complication rates have been estimated by case series, anecdotal reports, presentations at conferences and symposia and unpublished communications.[2] The available evidence to date indicates that the overall three-month post procedure complication rate is between 1.0% and 2.0%,[3,5,13] but it is expected to change as the evidence accumulates with longer follow-up.

REFERENCES

1. Ravina JH, Herbreteau D, Ciracu-Vigneron N, et al. (1995). Arterial embolization to treat uterine myomata. *Lancet* **346**: 671–2.
2. Burbank F & Hutchins FL (2000). Uterine artery occlusion by embolization or surgery for the treatment of fibroids: a unifying hypothesis-transient uterine ischemia. *J Am Assoc Gynecol Laparosc* **7**(4): S1–S49.
3. Hutchins FL, Worthington-Kirsch R & Berkowitz RP (1999). Selective uterine artery embolization as primary treatment for symptomatic leiomyomata uteri. *J Am Assoc Gynecol Laparosc* **6**(3): 279–84.
4. Hurst BS, Stackhouse DJ, Matthews ML & Marshburn PB (2000). Uterine artery embolization for symptomatic uterine myomas. *Fertil Steril* **74**(5): 855–69.
5. Goodwin SC, McLucas B, Lee M, et al. (1999). Uterine artery embolization for the treatment of uterine leiomyomata: midterm results. *J Vasc Interv Radiol* **10**: 1159–65.
6. Spies JB, Scialli AR, Jha RC, et al. (1999). Initial results from uterine fibroid embolization for symptomtic leiomyomata. *J Vasc Interv Radiol* **10**: 1149–59.
7. Spies JB, Ascher SA, Roth AR, Kim J, et al. (2001). Uterine artery embolization for leiomyomata. *Obstet Gynecol* **98**: 29–34.
8. Ravina JH, Ciracu-Vigneron NC, Aymard A, LeDref O & Merland JJ (1999). Uterine artery embolization for fibroid disease: results of a 6 year study. *Min Inv Ther Allied Technol* **8**: 441–7.
9. Worthington-Kirsch RL, Popky Gl, Hutchins FL (1998). Uterine artery embolization for the management of leiomyomas: quality-of-life assessment and clinical response. *Radiology* **208**: 625–9.
10. Goodwin SC & Walker WJ (1998). Uterine artery embolization for the treatment of uterine fibroids. *Curr Opin Obstet Gynecol* **10**: 315–20.
11. Dinarello CA & Bunn PA Jr (1997). Fever. *Semin Oncol* **24**: 288–98.
12. Boni RAH, Hebisch G, Huch A, et al. (1994). Multiple necrotic uterine leiomyomas causing severe puerperal fever: Ultrasound, CT, MRI, and histological findings. *J Comput Assist Tomogr* **18**: 828–31.
13. Walker W, Green A & Sutton C (1999). Bilateral uterine artery embolization for myoma: results, complications and failures. *Min Invas Ther Allied Technol* **8**: 449–54.
14. Forman RG, Reidy J, Nott V, Braude P (1999). Fibroids and Fertility. *Min Invas Ther Allied Technol* **8**: 415–19.
15. Vashisht A, Studd J, Carey A & Burn P (1999). Fatal septicaemia after fibroid embolization. *Lancet* **354**: 307–8.

16. Anonymous (2001). Antibiotic prophylaxis for gynecologic procedures. *ACOG Prac Bull* **23**: 109.

17. Siskin GP, Stainken BF, Dowling K, et al. (2000). Outpatient uterine artery embolization for symptomatic uterine fibroids: experience in 49 patients. *J Vasc Interv Radiol* **11**: 305–11.

18. Bradley E, Reidy J, Forman R, et al. (1998). Transcatheter uterine artery embolization to treat large uterine fibroids. *Br J Obstet Gynecol* **105**: 235–40.

19. Nicolic B, Spies JB, Lundsten MJ, et al. (2000). Patient radiation dose associated with uterine artery embolization. *Radiology* **214**: 121–5.

20. Stringer NH, Grant T, Park J & Oldham L (2000). Ovarian failure after uterine artery embolization for treatment of myomas. *J Am Assoc Gynecol Laparosc* **7**: 395–400.

21. Amato P & Roberts A (2001). Transient ovarian failure: a complication of uterine artery embolization. *Fertil Steril* **75**(2): 438–9.

22. Palmoba S, Sena T, Noia R, et al. (2001). Transdermal hormone replacement therapy in postmenopausal women with uterine leiomyomas. *Obstet Gynecol* **98**: 1053–8.

23. Pelage JP, LeDref O, Soyer P, et al. (2000). Fibroid related menorrhagia: treatment with super-elective embolization of the uterine arteries and midterm follow-up. *Radiology* **215**: 428–31.

24. Chrisman HB, Saker MB, Ryu RK, et al. (2000). The impact of uterine fibroid embolization on resumption of menses and ovarian function. *J Vasc Interv Radiol* **11**: 699–703.

25. Felemban A, Valenti D, Stein L & Tulandi T (2001). Spontaneous uterine restoration following uterine artery embolization and repeated expulsion of myomas. *J Am Assoc Gynecol Laparosc* **8**: 442–4.

26. McLucas B & Adler L (2000). Uterine artery embolization as therapy for myomata. *Infertil Reprod Med Clinics of N Am* **11**: 77–94.

27. De Iaco P, Muzzupapa G, Golfieri R, et al. (2002). A uterine wall defect after uterine artery embolization for symptomatic myomas. *Fertil Steril* **77**(1): 176–8.

28. De Iaco P, Golfieri R, Ghi T, et al. (2001) Uterine fistula induced by hysteroscopic resection of an embolized migrated fibroid: a rare complication after embolization of uterine fibroids. *Fertil Steril* **75**(4): 818–20.

29. Godfrey CD & Zbella EA (2001). Uterine necrosis after uterine artery embolization for leiomyoma. *Obstet Gynecol* **98**: 950–2.

30. Anonymous (2001). Myomas and reproductive function. A Practice Committee Report. *Am Soc Repro Med Educ Bull*.

31. Coronado GD, Marshall LM & Schwartz SM (2000). Complications in pregnancy, labor and delivery with uterine leiomyomas: A population-based study. *Obstet Gynecol* **95**: 764–9.

32. Ramzy AM, Sattor M, Amin Y, et al. (1998) Uterine myomata and outcome of assisted reproduction. *Hum Reprod* **13**: 198–202.

33. Eldar-Geva T, Meagher S, Healy DL, et al. (1998). Effect of intramural, subserosal and submucosal uterine fibroids on the outcome of assisted reproductive technology treatment. *Fertil Steril* **70**: 687–91.

34. Stancato-Pasik A, Mitty HA, Richard HM III & Eshka RN (1997). Obstetric embolotherapy: effect on menses and pregnancy. *Radiology* 791–3.

35. Ravina JH, Ciracu-Vigneron NC, Aymard A, et al. (2000). Pregnancy after embolization of uterine myoma: report of 12 cases. *Fertil Steril* **73**: 1241–3.

36. Leibshon S, D'Ablaing G, Mishell DR, Jr & Schlaerth JB (1990). Leiomyosarcoma in a series of hysterectomies performed for presumed uterine leiomyomas. *Am J Obstet Gynecol* **162**: 968–76.

37. Schwartz LB, Zaroin M, Concangiu ML, et al. (1998). Does pelvic magnetic resonance imaging differentiate among the histologic subtypes of uterine leiomyomata. *Fertil Steril* **70**: 580–7.

38. Barbazza R, Chiarelli S, Quintareli GF & Marchi R (1997). Role of fine-needle aspiration cytology in the pre-operative evaluation of smooth muscle tumors. *Diagn Cytopathol* **16**: 326–30.

39. Al-Badr Ahmed & Faught W (2001). Uterine artery embolization in undiagnosed uterine sarcoma. *Obstet Gynecol* **97**: 836–7.

40. Bergholt T, Eriksen L, Berendt N, Jacobsen M & Hertz JB (2001). Prevalence and risk factors of adenomyosis at hysterectomy. *Hum Reprod* **16**: 2418–21.

41. Tay SK & Bromwich N (1998). Outcome of hysterectomy for pelvic pain in perimenopausal women. *Aust NZ J Obstet Gynecol* **38**: 72–6.

42. Pelage JP, LeDref O, Soyer P, et al. (1999). Arterial anatomy of the female genital tract: variations and relevance to transcatheter embolization of the uterus. *Am J Roentgenol* **172**: 989–94.

43. Anonymous (2000). Prevention of deep thrombosis and pulmonary embolism. *ACOG Prac Bull* **21**: 1–10.

44. Chong YS, Fong YF & Ng SC (1998). Deep vein thrombosis in patients with large uterine myomata. *Obstet Gynecol* **92**(4): 707.

45. Bachmann GA (1990). Hysterectomy. A critical review. *J Reprod Med* **35**: 839–62.

16

Reproductive function after uterine artery embolization

Togas Tulandi

McGill University, Montreal, Quebec, Canada

Leiomyoma is the most common benign tumor occurring in the uterus and in the female pelvis. It is estimated that 25% of women over the age of 35 years have leiomyoma. Accordingly, not all women with myoma should be treated. As women continue to delay their childbearing until the third and fourth decades of life, leiomyoma will be encountered more frequently.

One of the newest treatments of uterine leiomyomata is uterine artery embolization (UAE).[1-7] The main purpose of UAE is to reduce the size of the myomata and to treat excessive uterine bleeding. In a review of 119 cases of UAE,[7] the authors reported that about 70% of the patients had an immediate cessation of menorrhagia and improvement of pain and pressure symptoms after the procedure. At six months follow-up, the total uterine volume decreased by 56% and the average diameter of the largest myoma decreased by 36%.

The purpose of this review is to evaluate the effects of UAE on reproductive function.

Uterine fibroids and fertility

The association between leiomyoma and infertility has been discussed for many years. Current evidence suggests that leiomyoma that deforms the uterine cavity decreases fertility. This could be related to poor implantation site or to impaired gamete transport. The best evidence came from the experience in in vitro fertilization (IVF).

Eldar-Geva et al.[8] compared the implantation and pregnancy rate of 88 women with uterine myoma (106 cycles) and 318 cycles of women without uterine myoma. The implantation rates of women with subserosal, intramural, and submucosal myoma were 15.1%, 6.4%, and 4.3%, whereas the pregnancy rates per transfer were 34.1%, 16.4%, and 10% respectively. Compared to the implantation and pregnancy rates of women without myoma (15.7% and 30.1%), these rates were significantly lower in women with intramural and submucous myoma, even when there was no deformation of the uterine cavity. In this study, pregnancy and implantation rates were not influenced by the presence of subserosal fibroids.

In another study, Surrey et al.[9] studied 319 IVF cycles in women with and without intramural myoma. All women had normal uterine cavity on hysteroscopy examination. There was no difference in the live birth rate among women with and without intramural myoma. The authors emphasized the need for hysteroscopy examination of the uterine cavity. Hart et al.,[10] on the other hand found that even in the presence of normal hysteroscopy and the size of intramural myoma of ≤ 5 cm, the pregnancy, implantation and ongoing pregnancy rates in women with myoma (23.3, 11.9 and 15.1) were significantly lower than in those without myoma (34.1, 20.2 and 28.3% respectively).

It seems clear that the presence of submucous myoma decreases fertility and removal of this type of myoma by hysteroscopy normalizes the pregnancy rate.[11,12] Fertility is not impaired by the presence of subserous myoma or intramural myoma that does not deform the uterine cavity. Distorted uterine cavity by intramural myoma can be corrected by myomectomy either by laparoscopy or by laparotomy. The results are similar.[13] In order to reduce the risks of uterine rupture, it is mandatory to perform multilayered suturing of the uterine incision. Only surgeons who are familiar with laparoscopic suturing should perform laparoscopic myomectomy.

Myomectomy, however, can lead to adhesion formation and periadnexal adhesions can lead to infertility. Adhesion formation after laparoscopic myomectomy is less than after myomectomy by laparotomy. The incidence of adhesions is approximately 48% after laparoscopic myomectomy and 70% after myomectomy by laparotomy. Whether UAE is associated with adhesion formation is unknown. It is possible that necrosis of a subserous myoma can also lead to adhesion formation.

Premature menopause

It is clear that UAE is an alternative treatment for women who do not wish to undergo a hysterectomy. However, following this procedure several women have become menopausal.[2–4,14,15] It seems that premature menopause following embolization occurs predominantly in the older aged group. This is due to embolization of the utero-ovarian collateral circulation compromising the blood supply to the ovaries.[15–17] Although perimenopausal women with their declining ovarian function tend to be more affected than younger women, it has also been reported in women younger than 40 years. The estimated risk is about 1%. Similar to others,[18] we have encountered permanent ovarian failure with severe menopausal symptoms in a 40-year-old woman immediately after UAE.

The risk of menopause is not confined to UAE. Laparoscopic coagulation of uterine arteries for the treatment of uterine myoma was associated with a premature menopause rate of 3.5%.[19] However, coagulation of the utero-ovarian collaterals in the ovarian ligament and the mesosalpinx was also done.

The occurrence of menopause in premenopausal women results in a decrease in estrogen concentration leading to the shrinkage of the myoma. Although this is beneficial, these women will need hormonal replacement therapy. Accordingly, it is important to carefully weigh the benefits and the risks of UAE in these women. Those who do not want to take the risk of possible early menopause can be offered a hysterectomy. On the other hand, myomectomy is a better alternative than UAE in women of the reproductive age who have not completed their family.

Ovarian function after UAE

In 2002 we evaluated ovarian function after UAE in 23 women with baseline serum follicle stimulating hormone (FSH) levels of <10 mIU/ml.[18] Day 3 serum FSH is an indirect measurement of ovarian reserve. As the number of follicles and quality decline with advancing age, serum basal FSH increases. This has been attributed to decreased production of inhibin by the ovaries. Day 3 serum FSH levels have been shown to be an accurate predictor of pregnancy rate after IVF.[20,21]

In agreement with a previous observation,[22] basal FSH levels increased following UAE (Figure 16.1). We also found a trend in increasing serum estradiol. These changes suggest a decreasing ovarian reserve after UAE.[20] The high estradiol levels indicate

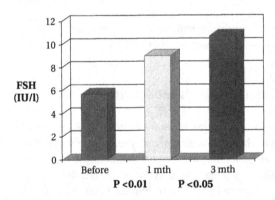

Figure 16.1. Serum follicle-stimulating hormone (FSH) levels before, one month and three months after uterine artery embolization.

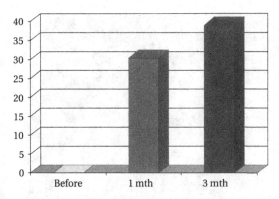

Figure 16.2. Percentage of women with serum follicle-stimulating hormone (FSH) >10 mIU/ml before, one month and three months after uterine artery embolization (UAE).

accelerated follicular recruitment in response to elevated FSH secretion. Increased level of >10 mIU/ml was encountered in seven women a month after the procedure and in nine women three months after UAE (Figure 16.2). The highest level was 22.8 mIU/ml a month after and 33.8 mIU/ml three months after the procedure. The declining ovarian reserve is also apparent in the tendency of decreasing number of antral follicles. Declining ovarian reserve is associated with poor pregnancy rate, but it is also related with recurrent pregnancy loss.[23]

Transient ovarian failure has been described.[24] The authors concluded that UAE might hasten ovarian failure. In our series, the FSH levels three months after embolization were higher than the levels at one month after UAE and the baseline levels in all patients.

In our institution, we offer UAE only to women with symptomatic myomata who have completed their family. Although they were not interested in conceiving, the decline in ovarian reserve in our patients is worrisome.

Pregnancy following uterine artery embolization

Pregnancies following UAE have been reported. Ravina[25] reported the largest number of pregnancies from one center. They noted 12 pregnancies in women aged 22–41 years. Of these, five resulted in a miscarriage and three in preterm deliveries. This high rate of miscarriage is concerning. Although it has not been reported, the decrease in uterine blood flow after UAE can also lead to intrauterine growth restriction. There is at least one report of intrauterine growth restriction after bilateral hypogastric artery ligation.[26] Regrowth of the myoma during pregnancy has been reported. Due to the possibility of expulsion of submucous and even intramural myoma leading to weakness of the uterine wall, UAE might carry the risk of uterine rupture.

UAE as an alternative to myomectomy in young women

If we could perform UAE without compromising the ovarian function, UAE would be able to replace myomectomy in young women. This would be especially helpful for women with intramural myoma that deforms the uterine cavity. Normalization of the uterine cavity might improve the implantation site and increases fertility. However, with the present technique, the risk of premature menopause and decreased ovarian function does not permit the use of UAE in reproductive aged women. Furthermore, necrosis of the uterus and a subserous myoma could cause adhesions that may further decrease fertility. UAE might also weaken the uterine wall leading to uterine rupture in pregnancy or labor.

In order not to embolize the utero-ovarian collaterals, one has to find the best candidates for UAE, perhaps women with a certain caliber of utero-ovarian collateral vessels, and changing the technique or the size of embolization particles. It appears that the smaller the particles, the deeper they reach into smaller vessels inside the muscle mass leading to a larger area of ischemia and infarction. Not only does it cause more pain, but it might also be associated with a higher incidence of infection and embolization of the utero-ovarian collaterals.

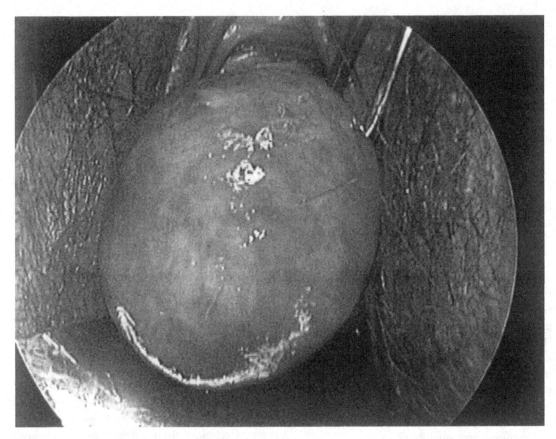

Figure 16.3. A prolapsing submucous myoma. See also color plates.

The commonly used size is 350–500 μ of polyvinyl alcohol.

Laparoscopic bipolar uterine artery coagulation as an alternative to UAE

In 2001, a group from Taiwan introduced laparoscopic bipolar coagulation of uterine vessels as an alternative to UAE.[27] Of the 87 patients who underwent the procedure, the average fibroid volume and uterine volume reductions were 76% and 46% respectively. The FSH levels in three patients was >30 mIU/ml postoperatively. However, their ages were 46, 48 and 53 years respectively. Two patients conceived after the procedure.

Because this procedure does not interrupt the utero-ovarian collaterals, it is unlikely that the treatment would be associated with premature ovarian failure or decreased ovarian function. Further study is needed to clarify this matter.

Conclusions

UAE is an alternative to hysterectomy in women who have completed their family. Report of pregnancy following UAE is anecdotal and the description of livebirth is still limited. Whether UAE carries the risks of adhesions and uterine rupture is unknown. Due to the concern of loss of ovarian function and risks of premature menopause, UAE should be reserved for women who do not desire future fertility. Further refinement of the technique and identification of women at risk of decreased ovarian function and premature menopause is needed.

REFERENCES

1. Ravina JH, Herbreteau D, Cigaru-Vigneron N, et al. (1995). Arterial embolization to treat uterine myomata. *Lancet* **346**: 671–2.

2. Bradley EA, Reidy JF, Forman RG, Jarosz J & Braude PR (1998). Transcatheter uterine artery embolization to treat large uterine fibroids. *Br J Obstet Gynaecol* **105**: 235–40.

3. Goodwin SC, McLucas B, Lee M, et al. (1999). Uterine artery embolization for the treatment of uterine leiomyomata midterm results. *J Vasc Interv Radiol* **10**: 1159–65.

4. Spies JB, Scialli AR, Jha RC, et al. (1999). Initial results from uterine artery embolization for symptomatic leiomyomata. *J Vasc Interv Radiol* **10**: 1149–57.

5. Hutchins FL Jr, Worthington-Kirsch R & Berkowitz RP (1999). Selective uterine artery embolization as primary treatment for symptomatic leiomyomata uteri. *J Am Assoc Gynecol Laparosc* **6**: 279–84.

6. Hurst BS, Stackhouse DJ, Matthews M & Marshburn PB (2000). Uterine artery embolization for symptomatic uterine myomas. *Fertil Steril* **74**: 855–69.

7. McLucas B & Adler L (2000). Uterine artery embolization as therapy for myomata. *Infertil Reprod Med Clinics of NAm* **11**: 77–94.

8. Eldar-Geva T, Meagher S, Healy DL, MacLachlan V, Breheny S & Wood C (1998). Effect of intramural, subserosal, and submucosal uterine fibroids on the outcome of assisted reproductive technology. *Fertil Steril* **70**: 687–91.

9. Surrey ES, Lietz AK & Schoolcraft WB (2001). Impact of intramural leiomyomata in patients with a normal endometrial cavity on in vitro fertilization-embryo transfer. *Fertil Steril* **75**: 405–10.

10. Hart R, Khalaf Y, Yeong CT, Seed P, Taylor A & Braude P (2001). A prospective controlled study of the effect of intramural uterine fibroids on the outcome of assisted conception. *Hum Reprod* **16**: 2411–17.

11. Farhi J, Ashkenazi J, Feldberg D, Dicker D, Orvieto R & Ben Rafael Z (1995). Effect of uterine leiomyomata on the results of in-vitro fertilization treatment. *Hum Reprod* **10**: 2576–8.

12. Pritts EA (2001). Fibroids and infertility: a systematic review of the evidence. *Obstet Gynecol Survey* **56**: 483–91.

13. Seracchioli R, Rossi S, Govoni F, Rossi E, Venturoli S, Bulletti C & Flamigni C (2000). Fertility and obstetric outcome after laparoscopic myomectomy of large myomata: a randomized comparison with abdominal myomectomy. *Hum Reprod* **15**: 2663–8.

14. Chrisman H, Saker M, Ryu R, et al. (2000). The impact of uterine fibroid embolization on resumption of menses and ovarian function. *J Vasc Interv Radiol* **11**: 699–703.

15. Stringer NH, Grant T, Park J & Oldham J (2000). Ovarian failure after uterine artery embolization for treatment of myomas. *J Am Assoc Gynecol Laparosc* **7**: 395–400.

16. Matson M, Nicholson A & Belli AM (2000). Anastomoses of the ovarian and uterine arteries: a potential pitfall and cause of failure of uterine embolization. *Cardiovasc Intervent Radiol* **23**: 393–6.

17. Tulandi T, Sammour A, Valenti D & Stein L (2001). Uterine artery embolization and utero-ovarian collateral. *J Am Assoc Gynecol Laparosc* **8**: 474.

18. Tulandi T, Sammour A, Valenti D, Child TJ, Seti L & Tan SL (2002). Ovarian reserve after uterine artery embolization for leiomyomata. *Fertil Steril* **178**: 197–8.

19. Liu WM (2000). Laparoscopic bipolar coagulation of uterine vessels to treat symptomatic leiomyomas. *J Am Assoc Gynecol Laparosc* **7**: 125–9.

20. Scott RT, Toner JP, Muasher SJ, et al. (1989). Follicle stimulating hormone levels on day 3 are predictive of in vitro fertilization outcome. *Fertil Steril* **51**: 651–4.

21. Magarelli PC, Pearstone AC & Buyalos R (1996). Discrimination between chronological and ovarian age in infertile women aged 35 and older: predicting pregnancy using basal follicle stimulating hormone, age and number of ovulation induction/intrauterine insemination cycles. *Hum Reprod* **11**: 1214–19.

22. Spies JB, Roth AR, Gonsalves SM & Murphy-Skrzyniarz KM (2001). Ovarian function after uterine artery embolization for leiomyomata: assessment with use of serum follicle stimulating hormone. *J Vasc Interv Radiol* **12**: 437–42.

23. Trout SW & Seifer DB (2000). Do women with unexplained recurrent pregnancy loss have higher day 3 serum FSH and estradiol values? *Fertil Steril* **74**: 335–7.

24. Amato P & Roberts AC (2001). Transient ovarian failure: a

complication of uterine artery embolization. *Fertil Steril* **75**: 438–9.

25. Ravina JH, Cigaru-Vigneron N, Aymard A, Le Dref O & Merland JJ (2000). Pregnancy after embolization of uterine myoma: report of 12 cases. *Fertil Steril* **73**: 1241–3.

26. Morikawa S & Tamakizawa H (1986). Delivery of small date infant following bilateral ligation of iliac arteries. *Asia Oceania J Obstet Gynecol* **12**: 213–16.

27. Liu WM, Ng HT, Wu YC, Yen YK & Yuan CC (2001). Laparoscopic bipolar coagulation of uterine vessels: a new method for treating symptomatic fibroids. *Fertil Steril* **75**: 417–22.

17

Reasons and prevention of embolization failure

Bruce McLucas

UCLA Medical Center, Los Angeles, CA, USA

This chapter will examine the failures of uterine artery embolization (UAE) in our center. The overall results of UAE and our standard to define failures have been discussed in Chapter 14. In short, these standards are minimal or no shrinkage, no relief of symptoms, and hysterectomy.[1,2] Here, we will also discuss technical failures and failures to achieve fertility.

Excluded patients

In our practice, we perform endoscopic evaluations of the uterus, as well as taking into account the possible contraindication or factors that may lead to failure. We exclude patients prior to embolization using the scheme outlined in the Chapter 14. Prevention of failure starts with selecting the correct procedure. We have excluded six patients with gynecologic malignancy. Twelve patients who presented with acute uterine hemorrhage and were embolized prior to endoscopic evaluation on an emergency basis were evaluated with endoscopy after embolization. One of these patients was discovered to have a malignancy and was referred for a definitive therapy. We also excluded 22 patients with atypical endometrial hyperplasia and eight patients with acute pelvic infection.

Definition of failure

Minimal shrinkage

Shrinkage alone is not a sole criterion of success. Later in this chapter, we will analyze patients who presented with uterine shrinkage of 50%, but they could not be categorized into the success group.

Nonetheless, others have reported success as long as there is shrinkage in the size of the fibroid. To date, we have embolized a total of 595 patients. Of these, 301 patients had an ultrasound evaluation approximately six months after the UAE, and recorded an average uterine shrinkage of 44.8%. They also achieved an average of 31.4% shrinkage of the largest myoma. We found 29 patients who experienced shrinkage of ≤10% and we considered this minimal shrinkage as a failure.

No relief of symptoms

Before UAE, we ask the patients to describe the three symptoms commonly associated with myomata – menorrhagia (or postmenopausal bleeding), pressure symptoms, and pain. Although somewhat arbitrary, we categorize patients into three groups: mild, moderate, and severe. At six months, and throughout the study period, we asked the same questions (Table 17.1).

Patients with persistent or worsening symptoms are categorized into the failure group. Using this criterion, we encountered failure in 13 patients. We found that a number of patients with pedunculated subserous myomata reported abdominal pain about a year after the procedure. On laparoscopy, we found that the pedunculated myoma was covered by adhesions (Figure 17.1a,b, see also color plates). We speculated that the embolized myoma became necrotic leading to adhesion formation. Today, we

Table 17.1. Results of symptom questionnaires before and six months following uterine artery embolization

Severity of symptom	Bleeding	Pain	Pressure
Pre-procedure			
Mild	54	39	4
Moderate	148	108	36
Severe	392	448	554
6 month follow-up			
None	116	128	6
Mild	442	449	585
Moderate	29	13	2
Severe	8	5	2

offer such patients UAE followed immediately by laparoscopic myomectomy. This approach leads to a bloodless myomectomy and might decrease adhesion formation.

Hysterectomy

We consider any patient who underwent an unplanned hysterectomy after embolization to be a failure. In our series, we encountered 31 patients. Of the total 31 patients, 21 underwent hysterectomy for diagnosis not associated with myomata. Nonetheless, these patients were included in the failure group.

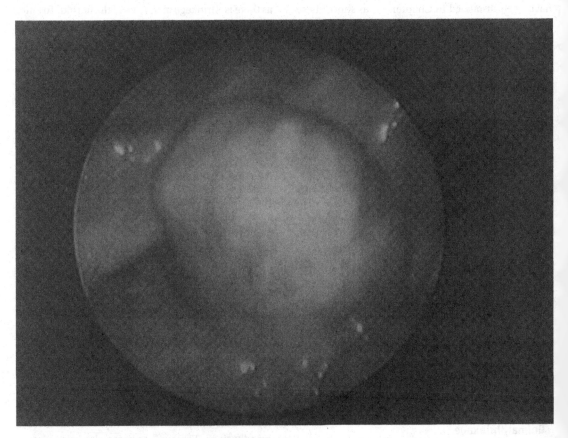

Figure 17.1a. Subserosal fibroid prior to embolization. See color plates.

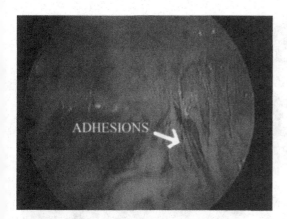

Figure 17.1b. Same patient as for 17.1a two years later. See also color plates.

Eleven (36%) of the hysterectomized patients had had adenomyosis, suggesting that this condition is refractory to embolization.[3] When we evaluated our results three years after embolization, we found no further increase in the incidence of hysterectomy. There appears to be a higher immediate failure leading to a hysterectomy.

Two patients had an infection within a month after UAE, and underwent a hysterectomy. One of these patients had not been screened with endoscopy prior to embolization.

The pathology report on the hysterectomy specimen revealed acute and chronic salpingitis. It is possible that the patient had an underlying infection at the time of UAE. A second patient suffered from persistent fever and pain after embolization. At the time of hysterectomy, we found extrusion of the intramural myoma through the serosa, presumably by gas forming organisms (Figure 17.2, see also color plates).

Note that of a total of 50 000 UAE procedures, one death has been reported. This was due to failed recognition and management of an infection.[4] Whereas post-embolization syndrome is the more likely cause for temperature elevation and fever, physicians must aggressively evaluate any patient with a possible infectious process. An abscess will be clearly visible on computed tomography (CT) scan (Figure 17.3) and the treatment is hysterectomy.

Despite shrinkage of >50%, six patients were included in the failure group. Two patients had no relief of symptoms, and four underwent a hysterectomy.

Analysis of failure group

In our failure group, 29 patients had uterine shrinkage of less that 10%, 13 had persistent or worsening symptoms, and 31 underwent hysterectomy following embolization. Factors associated with failures are large myomas (>8.5 cm) and uterine size in our upper 10 percentile. Operator experience does not seem to play a role in failure. In our group, only one physician had a higher failure rate in the first 20 patients.

Technical failure

Our technical failures were described previously.[5] We define technical failure as the inability to embolize both uterine arteries. We encountered 19 patients with technical failure. Of these, the operator experienced technical difficulties in 10 patients. In the remaining nine patients, anomaly of the uterine arteries was encountered including no obvious uterine artery on one side.

In our practice, we offer another UAE by another physician if the first failure is due to operator's difficulties. Ten patients underwent a second embolization for this indication. Eight of the 10 patients underwent UAE successfully on the second attempt. Their average uterine shrinkage was 28%.

Treatment failures

There are three types of patient who would benefit from repeat UAE. They are patients who failed immediately following UAE, patients who failed shortly after UAE, and patients who showed initial success but later experienced a return of symptoms. We previously reported unsuccessful attempts to re-enter the uterine artery after embolization with polyvinyl alcohol (PVA) particles.[6] We have since reexamined

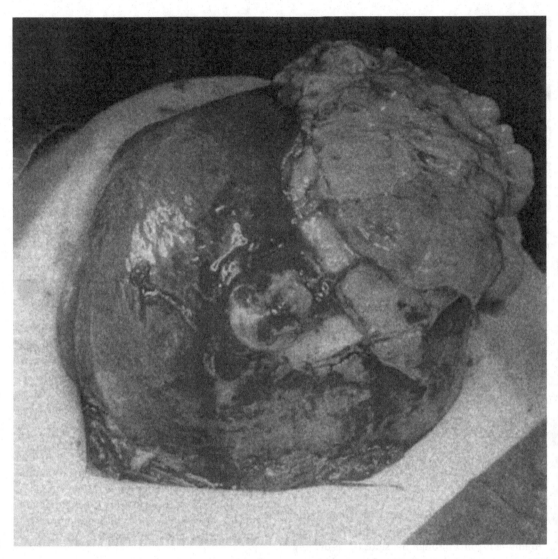

Figure 17.2. Extrusion of infected intramural fibroid following hysterectomy. See also color plates.

our earlier conclusion. The following case report is illustrative.

A 46-year-old woman underwent a successful UAE using 700-μ embospheres. Due to persistent heavy menstruation and the magnetic resonance imaging (MRI) findings of slight increase in the size of the uterus and myomata, she underwent another UAE 90 days later. At the time of the second UAE, flow was seen in both uterine arteries. Both arteries were again embolized. Since then, the patient has had one menstrual cycle, which was normal.

A third group of patients are those who underwent embolization with initial good results. Then, the symptoms return. We have encountered four patients in this group. Note that in the presence of deep adenomyosis, a second procedure might not be useful. Two patients had a repeat UAE in this category (Figure 17.4).

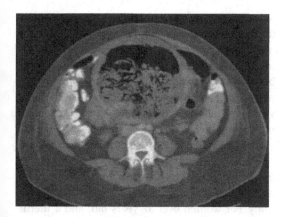

Figure 17.3. CT Scan post-embolization diagnosing uterine abscess.

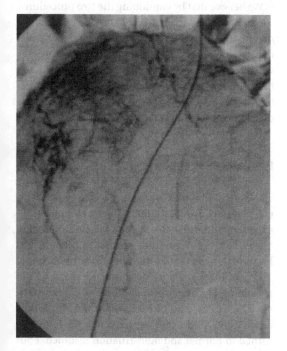

Figure 17.4. Angiography from repeat embolization demonstrating blood supply to the uterus from the left ovarian artery.

Another case was a 48-year-old woman with a 20 weeks' gestational age uterus who experienced an acute uterine bleeding and a hematocrit of 17%. The patient was treated with emergency UAE using 300-μ

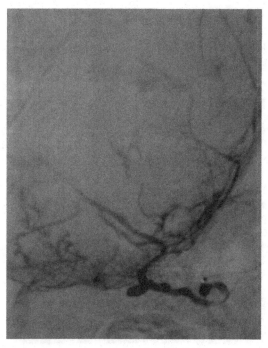

Figure 17.5a. Left uterine artery prior to embolization.

particles of PVA. The endpoint of the procedure was complete stasis (Figure 17.5a,b). Post-embolization, the patient was examined by hysteroscopy and found to have no malignancy or deep adenomyosis. The patient did well for the first four years after the procedure. The total uterine volume decreased from 1718 ml to 339 ml in March 2001. Over the same period, the largest myoma decreased in size from 16.3 cm to 5.5 cm. The patient's symptoms abated until the spring of 2002. Subsequently, she again experienced acute and severe uterine bleeding. Increased uterine volume and myoma diameter were noted on ultrasound. Her hematocrit was 25% and a repeat UAE was performed. At the time of this second procedure, flow was seen through both uterine arteries. It seemed that recanalization had occurred. The uterine arteries were again embolized, this time with 500-μ embosphere particles. The ovarian arteries were visualized and found not to supply the uterus. The patient has since not experienced further symptoms.

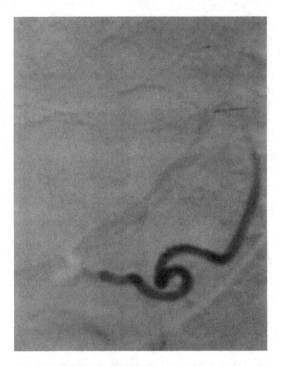

Figure 17.5b. Complete stasis in same artery after uterine artery embolization.

Each of these three categories represent patients whose UAE was successful, and experienced no change or recurrence of symptoms. Based on the success of these repeat procedures, we now offer our patients a repeat procedure for either persistent symptoms or failure to shrink six month after UAE.

Pregnancy after uterine artery embolization

The effects of UAE on fertility are still unclear.[7] In our practice, we only accept patients for UAE if they experience symptoms such as menorrhagia or pain and pressure. We have encountered a patient who suffered two mid-trimester losses after UAE. The initial size of her uterus prior to embolization was 2500 ml. Her first conception occurred 15 months post-procedure. At 16 gestational weeks, she reported amniotic fluid leakage and uterine contractions.

Subsequently, she miscarried. Hysteroscopy performed after the event revealed a sessile submucous myoma protruding into the endometrial cavity. The uterine volume decreased to 1985 ml a year after embolization. The patient reported adequate symptom relief. However, another miscarriage occurred one year later. Subsequently, she underwent abdominal myomectomy.

We have modified our treatment recommendations for women who desire fertility. For women with a uterus of greater than 16-week size, we recommend a UAE followed immediately by abdominal myomectomy. For women over 37 years old, and a uterus larger than 12 weeks in size, we recommend the same combined procedures.

We believe that by combining the two procedures we subject the patients to a 1% risk of premature menopause. On the benefit side, the patient will not experience any regrowth, a phenomenon that will affect 30% of myomectomy patients.[8] Also, the hemostasis in the recently embolized uterus is much better. We have experienced negligible blood loss during myomectomy after UAE.

Premature menopause

Here, we summarize our group's experience with early menopause. Of the 595 patients embolized, 47 experienced a rise in their serum follicle stimulating hormone (FSH) level from normal to menopausal levels within the first 12 months after embolization. Thirty of these patients were over 45 years. Of the remaining 17 patients under 45 years, eight experienced an initial rise in FSH within the 12 months after embolization, and subsequently the levels returned to normal and menstruation resumed. Four patients with an initial rise in FSH were lost to follow up. A remaining five patients under 45 years suffered a rise in FSH, and their postmenopausal symptoms persisted. Thus, in our population the rate of premature menopause is 0.8%.

It has been postulated that this complication is due to reflux of particles around the tip of the catheter into the ovarian artery.[9] In January 1999, we changed our group's policy of complete stasis as an endpoint to a less aggressive embolization. Since the change in our practice, two patients had premature menopause after UAE.

Discussion

We are comfortable with our definition of failure, which encompasses both symptom relief and shrinkage. With shrinkage alone, several patients who met the success criterion ultimately underwent hysterectomy.

We have demonstrated that patients who suffered a technical failure because of operator inability to cannulate the uterine artery could be offered a repeat procedure with good chance of success. A different operator will often make a difference to the outcome. Often, sufficient change in hemodynamics of flow after a one-sided embolization will facilitate catheterization of the opposite artery at a later date.

Our group has experienced an arterial tear requiring vascular repair, and thus preventing the possibility of embolization. Patients should be counseled about this small risk.

We have reported two patients who suffered an immediate infection, resulting in hysterectomy. It seems that one of the patients had a pre-existing infection. The second patient had a uterus of 28 gestational weeks. She underwent UAE early in our series when complete stasis was the objective. The patient required 10.75 vials of PVA, compared to the average of 3.62 vials per embolization. We have since altered our endpoint of embolization. We now use fewer particles in the large uterus and relied on larger particles and gelfoam to achieve the desired anoxic state.

A case report of uterine necrosis has been published.[10] We agree that this is an example of infection and necrosis after embolization.[11]

MRI studies have shown that the uterus reperfuses rapidly after UAE.[12] When we performed a laparoscopic myomectomy immediately after UAE, the uterus was initially blue and cyanotic. By the end of a one-hour procedure, the pink color of healthy myometrium returned.

Concerning fertility, we have modified our recommendations based on our experience. We recommend UAE as a stand-alone procedure for women of <35 years of age and with a uterus of <16 gestational weeks. We believe that the risk of premature menopause in this population is virtually nonexistent. Embolization offers patients desiring fertility a single treatment therapy for successful term pregnancies. Other benefits of embolization in this group include no recurrences of myomata, ability to deliver vaginally, and absence of adhesion formation.[13]

For patients >35 years of age, with a uterus of >16 gestational weeks, we now recommend a UAE immediately followed by abdominal myomectomy. The only patients experiencing pregnancy loss after UAE were in this size category. Following UAE we recommend a six-month waiting period prior to conception.

In the older patients, we recommend the combined procedure. By performing myomectomy after UAE, the surgeon will experience a near bloodless surgery. This will decrease the need for blood products, and decrease the conversion from myomectomy to hysterectomy.

We concur with others who caution against treatment of myomata for the sake of infertility alone.[14] We only treat patients whose myomata are symptomatic. Pedunculated subserous myomas may be a nidus for adhesion formation.[15] This may be avoided by performing a laparoscopic myomectomy immediately after UAE. Pedunculated submucous myomata have a high expulsion rate.[16,17] This should not be considered as failure. Such expulsion may be easily treated with a vaginal myomectomy.[1]

So, we are left with the questions, What is the failure rate of UAE? Is there a "base rate" of failure for UAE? Looking at our failure group, we note the correlation between the myoma size and failure. Perhaps very large myomas have a different response to anoxia, with a smaller shrinkage rate. In our group of patients who underwent hysterectomy, a large proportion of women had a larger uterus prior to UAE. Even with >50% shrinkage, a uterus greater than 24 weeks gestation size will still be quite sizable after UAE.

Of our patients, 22 underwent a hysterectomy due to coexistence of adenomyosis and myomas.[18] The incidence of premature menopause is 0.8%. With less aggressive embolization techniques, we encountered only two women with premature menopause after UAE.

We believe that patients will experience a successful delivery after embolization if they are <35 years of age and have a uterus of < sixteen weeks in size prior to UAE. Otherwise, a combination UAE and myomectomy would be a better alternative.

Embolization has been performed in several settings by our group, and by several different operators. The results are remarkably similar. The reproducibility of UAE has been shown worldwide. We have followed a group of 40 patients for more than five years. These patients have experienced continued uterine shrinkage, and no new myomata have been reported. The hysterectomy rate among this group is extremely low (5%). We are comfortable offering UAE as a permanent solution to patients with symptomatic myomata.

REFERENCES

1. McLucas B, Adler L & Perrella R (2001). Uterine fibroid embolization: nonsurgical treatment for symptomatic fibroids. *J Am Coll Surg* **192**: 95–105.

2. McLucas B, Alder L & Perrella R (1999). Predictive factors for success in uterine fibroid embolisation. *Min Invas Ther & Allied Technol* **8**: 429–32.

3. McLucas B, Perrella R & Adler L (2002). Embolization for the treatment of adenomyosis. (Letter.) *Am J Roentgenol* **178**: 1028–29.

4. Vashisht A, Studd J, Carey A & Burn P (1999). Fatal septicaemia after fibroid embolisation. *Lancet* **354**: 307–8.

5. McLucas B, Reed RA, Goodwin S, Rappaport A, Adler L,

Perrella R & Dalrymple J (2002). Outcomes following unilateral uterine artery embolisation. *Br J Radiol* **75**: 122–6.

6. Binkert C, Andrews R & Kaufman J (2001). Utility of non-selective abdominal aortography in demonstrating ovarian artery collaterals in patients undergoing uterine artery embolization for fibroids. *J Vasc Interv Radiol* **12**: 841–5.

7. Abulafia O & Sherer DM (1999). Transcatheter of uterine artery embolization for the management of symptomatic uterine leiomyomas. *Obstet Gynecol Surv* **12**: 745–53.

8. McLucas B & Adler L (2001). Uterine fibroid embolization compared with myomectomy. *Int J Gynaecol Obstet* **74**: 297–9.

9. Spies JB, Roth AR, Gonsalves SM & Murphy-Skrzyniarz KM (2001). Ovarian function after uterine artery embolization for leiomyomata: assessment with use of serum follicle stimulating hormone assay. *J Vasc Interv Radiol* **12**: 437–42.

10. Godfrey CD & Zbella EA (2001). Uterine necrosis after uterine artery embolization for leiomyoma. *Obstet Gynecol* **98**: 950–2.

11. Pelage JP, Walker WJ & Dref OL (2002). Uterine necrosis after uterine artery embolization for leiomyoma. (Letter.) *Obstet Gynecol* **99**: 676–7.

12. Katsumori T, Nakajima K & Hanada Y (1999). MR imaging of a uterine myoma after embolization. *Am J Roentgenol* **172**: 248–9.

13. McLucas B, Goodwin S, Adler L, Rappaport A, Reed R & Perella R (2001). Pregnancy following uterine fibroid embolization. *Int J Gynaecol Obstet* **74**: 1–7.

14. Gehlbach D, Sousa RC, Carpenter SE & Rock JA (1993). Abdominal myomectomy in the treatment of infertility. *Int J Gynecol Obstet* **40**: 45–50.

15. McLucas B, Goodwin & Adler L (1998). Adhesion formation following embolization. *Min Invas Ther & Allied Technol* (Abstract.) **7**(Supp 1): 42.

16. Abbara S, Spies JB, Scialli AR, Jha RC, Lage JM & Nikolic B (1999). Transcervical expulsion of a fibroid as a result of uterine artery embolization for leiomyomata. *J Vasc Intervent Radiol* **10**: 409–11.

17. Berkowitz RP, Hutchins FL & Worthington-Kirsch RL (1999). Vaginal expulsion of submucosal fibroids after uterine artery embolization. *J Reprod Med* **44**: 373–6.

18. Carlson KJ, Nichols DH & Schiff I (1993). Indications for hysterectomy. *N Engl J Med* **328**: 856.

Future of embolization and other therapies from gynecologic perspectives

Francis L. Hutchins, Jr.

Annapolis, Maryland, USA

Introduction

Since the first reports of uterine artery embolization (UAE) for treatment of fibroids,[1-3] the technique has been met with more enthusiasm by radiologists and patients than by gynecologists. This is quite understandable since this new procedure threatens the traditional exclusivity of gynecologists over the treatment of uterine leiomyomas. In a fee-based healthcare system, embolotherapy constitutes a direct economic threat to gynecologists.

As a consequence, the Society for Cardiovascular and Interventional Radiology (SCVIR) in its October 2000 survey reported that only 10 501 UAEs had been performed worldwide, with 8644 in the United States.[4] These are extremely low numbers considering that in the United States at least 200 000 hysterectomies are performed each year for fibroids. It suggests that this highly effective treatment is underutilized because of the turf issues between gynecologists and radiologists. It is clear that much of the future of UAE will be shaped by this struggle.

The advent of UAE is part of a continuum of minimally invasive procedures that have been gaining favor over the past 10–20 years. This trend, which has brought operative laparoscopy and operative hysteroscopy, will continue and impact on the future use of UAE. In a similar fashion, the trend towards the use of medical therapies such as gonadotropin-releasing hormone (GnRH) agonists will also influence the future of embolotherapy for fibroids.

Who will perform it?

As long as UAE remains as a therapy for fibroids there will be a question as to whether it will continue to be performed by interventional radiologists or whether gynecologists will be trained to perform it much as interventional cardiologists and vascular surgeons have been trained to perform the interventional techniques specific to their specialties. There appear to be several problems with this concept as was pointed out by Worthington-Kirsch.[5]

- Embolotherapy is a unique skill of those with extensive experience with angiography.
- In other specialties, training is integrated into the core-training program followed by one to three years of concentrated fellowship.
- Embolotherapy requires an integrated knowledge of fluoroscopy, radiation dosages and angiography.

Thus for the gynecologist to acquire the necessary skill, it will require at least two to three years of training and experience. This time commitment is certainly possible but would best be accomplished through a cooperative program between radiology and obstetrics and gynecology (OB/GYN) beginning in residency followed by a fellowship. Optimistically the area of interventional OB/GYN could develop out of this. Such a specialty would not only perform embolotherapy for fibroids and uterine bleeding but a broad range of imaging techniques to perform procedures such as drainage of cysts and abscesses, tubal catheterizations, etc. Because of the time necessary to become skilled, it is unlikely that gynecologists will perform embolotherapy routinely in the near future. In the present climate, it is equally unlikely that radiologists will cooperate with a training program for their "competitors."

Is it possible that interventional radiologists will train to care for fibroids? This is unlikely as well. To care for women with fibroids requires not only the ability to diagnose their presence but a thorough knowledge of female reproductive medicine including the relationship of fibroids to reproductive failure. In addition, one must be familiar with the differential diagnosis of abnormal uterine bleeding, pelvic pain, and the pelvic mass. Such knowledge represents a large part of what is contained in the 18 months of the gyn portion of an OB/GYN residency. It is unlikely that an interventional radiologist would devote this much time to develop a skill set in only one of the many diseases which they treat.

This brings us back to where we started with the radiologist dependent on the gynecologist to refer liberally women with fibroids when UAE is an appropriate option. The only possible stimulus to such referral would be a tightening of reimbursement for gynecologic surgery that would completely discourage the performance of surgery. This is not intended to overlook the fact that patients should be referred for UAE because it is the right thing to do. On the contrary, it is prompted by the knowledge that up to the present time this ethical incentive, apparently, has proven to be insufficient in most cases since relatively few women have been treated with UAE.

A final option would be the development of methods for achieving the same results as UAE through methodologies that can be performed totally or partially by gynecologists. As will be discussed later in this chapter, this option is being pursued.

Pregnancy

At present, as discussed in Chapter 12, there is a paucity of quality information regarding the impact of uterine artery occlusion on future pregnancy. Nevertheless, there are numerous reports of successful pregnancy after occluding the uterine arteries. Compromised uterine perfusion leading to placental insufficiency and fetal growth restriction is a serious concern. However, this complication has never been observed in post-UAE patients. Magnetic resonance imaging (MRI) studies of the uterus post-occlusion[6] have demonstrated that collateral circulation restores perfusion of the myometrium by one week after occlusion. Another concern could be that the myometrium may be weakened by the acute degeneration of the fibroids. Walker et al.[7] reported a case of uterine rupture after UAE. This rupture occurred early in the experience and may have been due to the very small particle size they were using for embolization. A literature search failed to identify either a similar report or a report of rupture during pregnancy post-embolization.

A final concern is premature ovarian failure. This seems primarily to be a problem in women over 45 years of age.[5,8] It is quite likely that these problems will be resolved either through alterations of technique or patient selection. That being the case uterine artery occlusion (UAO) could be useful in young women with modest myomas who do not plan pregnancy in the near future because of education or career goals. These women could be treated prophylactically to protect against excessive growth of the tumors that might threaten successful pregnancy in the future.

Embolization or occlusion

Since UAE began to be accepted as a viable treatment for myomas, there has been a desire to find a methodology that achieves the same results by using a technique that gynecologists can perform and for which they can be reimbursed. An example of this is laparoscopic uterine artery ligation or coagulation that has been reported to have similar results to UAE.[9–11] It is unlikely that the laparoscopic approach will prove to be truly competitive with UAE as it requires:

• surgical entry into the abdominal cavity;
• major anesthesia;

• more skill than most gynecologists possess.

It is, however, an important landmark in that it establishes the principal that UAO by any means is as effective in treating fibroids. This expands substantially the possibilities that can be explored in searching for the gynecologic alternative to UAE.

Recognizing this fact, Vascular Control Systems, Inc. in California, for whom I have been a consultant, has been pursuing a method where the uterine arteries can be occluded vaginally, a route that is very familiar to gynecologists. It is likely that similar simplified approaches will be explored, eventually providing the much sought gynecologic alternative.

Where will it be performed

Currently, all UAEs are performed in a hospital setting with discharge the same day or the following morning. Originally all patients were hospitalized. As pain control techniques continue to improve it will be possible for patients to be discharged shortly after the procedure. As the technique of UAO advances, even in its embolization form, the procedure will move to free standing outpatient facilities. When this occurs UAO will replace the need for surgery in the majority of women with fibroids.

Future alternatives

Pharmacologic therapy[12] will continue to evolve. This will offer both long-term and short-term relief of fibroid symptoms. Medications such as mifepristone that have a tumor suppression effect and without producing estrogen deficiency syndrome will likely have broad use in some patients.

In recent years, the unraveling of the genetics of leiomyomas has occurred.[13,14] This new understanding will enable gene therapy to potentially replace many other treatments for myomas. Niu et al.[15] have already reported a novel experiment using gene therapy. They were able to transfect the thymidine kinase producing capability from herpes simplex virus to rat leiomyoma cells in culture. This resulted in the leiomyoma cells being susceptible to gangciclovir, an antiviral drug. These altered cells also produced a "bystander effect" which caused death of nearby normal leiomyoma cells. Such experiments suggest the future possibility, if not likelihood, that gene therapy for destroying fibroids will become available.

As the genetics of myomas becomes better known it may become feasible to prevent fibroids through a variety of mechanisms obviating the need for treatment completely.

Conclusions

It is my belief that the turf battles between gynecologists and interventional radiologists will be resolved in the future. Eventually the need for even the minimally invasive treatments such as UAO will be replaced by improved medical therapies and genetic manipulations. Such developments could dramatically alter the practice of gynecology from a surgically oriented specialty to one which is largely nonsurgical.

REFERENCES

The publisher has used its best endeavours to ensure that the URLs for external websites referred to in this book are correct and active at the time of going to press. However, the publisher has no responsibility for the websites and can make no guarantee that a site will remain live or that the content is or will remain appropriate.

1. Ravina JH, Aymard A, Ciraru-Vigneron N, et al. (1998). Embolisation artérielle particulaire: un nouveau traitement des hémorragies des léiomyomes utérins. *Presse Med* **27**: 299–303.
2. Goodwin SC, Vedantham S, McLucas B, et al. (1997). Uterine artery embolization for treatment of uterine fibroids: Results of a pilot study. *J Vasc Interv Rad* **8**: 517–26.
3. Hutchins FL, Worthington-Kirsch RL & Berkowitz RP (1999). Selective uterine artery embolization as primary treatment for symptomatic leiomyomata uteri: a review of 305 consecutive cases. *J Am Assoc Gynecol Laparosc* **6**(3): 279–84.
4. UAE survey results available on SCVIR website at www.scvir.org/misc/uaesrvrt.htm

5. Hutchins FL & Worthington-Kirsch R (2000). Embolotherapy for myoma induced menorrhagia. *Obstet Gynecol Clin North Am* **27**(2): 397–405.

6. Burbank F & Hutchins FL (2000). Uterine artery occlusion by embolization or surgery for treatment of fibroids: a unifying hypothesis-transient uterine ischemia. *J Am Assoc Gynecol Laparosc* **7**(4 Suppl): S1–S49.

7. Walker W, Green A & Sutton C (1999). Bilateral uterine artery embolization for myomata: results, complications and failures. *Min Invas Ther & Allied Technol* **8**(6): 449–54.

8. Spies JB, Roth AR, Gonsalves SM & Murphy-Skrzyniarz KM (2001). Ovarian function after uterine artery embolization for leiomyomata: assessment with use of serum follicle stimulating hormone assay. *J Vasc Interv Radiol* **12**(4): 437–42.

9. Liu WM (2000). Laparoscopic bipolar coagulation of uterine vessels to treat symptomatic leiomyomas. *J Am Assoc Gynecol Laparosc* **7**(1): 125–9.

10. Lee PI, Chang YK, Yoon JB & Chi YS (2000). Preliminary experience with uterine artery ligation of symptomatic leiomyomas. *J Am Assoc Gynecol Laparosc* **6**(3): 125–9.

11. Liu WM, Ng HT, Wu YC, et al. (2001). Laparoscopic bipolar coagulation of uterine arteries in treating symptomatic uterine fibroids. *Fertil Steril* **75**(2): 417–22.

12. Chavez NF & Stewart EA (2001). Medical treatment of uterine fibroids. *Clin Obstet Gynecol* **44**(2): 372–84.

13. Ligon Ah & Morton CC (2000). Genetics of leiomyomata. *Genes Chromosomes Cancer* **28**(3): 235–45.

14. Li S & McLachlan JA (2001). Estrogen associated genes in leiomyoma. *Ann NY Academy Sci* **948**: 112–20.

15. Niu H, Simari RD, Zimmerman EM, et al. (1998). Nonviral vector-mediated thymidine kinase gene transfer and gangciclovir treatment in leiomyoma cells. *Obstet Gynecol* **91** (5 Pt 1): 735–40.

19

The future of fibroid embolotherapy: a radiological perspective

Robert L. Worthington-Kirsch[1] and Wendy J. Landow[2]

[1]Philadelphia College of Osteopathic Medicine, Pennsylvania, USA
[2]Society of Interventional Radiology, Virginia, USA

Background

Symptomatic fibroids are a major health concern for women. An estimated 177 000 to 366 000 hysterectomies and approximately 35 000 myomectomies are performed each year in the United States for this problem.[1] In addition, many women receive medical treatment for fibroids and many others suffer symptoms but never undergo treatment. Uterine artery embolization (UAE) offers great promise as a treatment for symptomatic fibroids.

The utility of embolotherapy for fibroid disease was a serendipitous discovery made by the French gynecologist Jacques Ravina and his colleagues at Hopital Lariboisiere in Paris.[2,3] As such, UAE for fibroids is merely a new indication for a technique that has been used successfully for several decades for the endovascular treatment of female genital tract bleeding of arterial origin. The safety and efficacy of uterine artery embolotherapy for post-surgical and post-partum hemorrhage has been established since the procedure was first reported for these indications in 1979.[4,5] More recently, the safety and efficacy of uterine embolotherapy has been demonstrated for the treatment of cervical ectopic pregnancy and in the management of some abnormalities of placentation.[6,7]

The current literature on UAE for fibroids has already demonstrated that it is a safe and effective treatment for fibroid disease, at least in the short to mid term.[8–12] In the United States and Canada there have been several unsuccessful attempts to conduct randomized prospective studies comparing UAE to either myomectomy or hysterectomy. These have failed because patients were unwilling to be randomized between UAE and a major abdominal surgery. A small-randomized trial of UAE vs. hysterectomy was conducted in Spain, but has not yet been published.[13] There are currently two industry-supported comparative cohort studies of UAE vs. surgery (one vs. myomectomy, the other vs. hysterectomy) in progress. The initial results of one of these have been presented,[14] showing UAE to be safe and effective when compared to hysterectomy.

The Cardiovascular and Interventional Radiology Research and Education Foundation (CIRREF) and the Society of Interventional Radiology (SIR), in co-operation with the Duke Clinical Research Institute (DCRI), have established the UAE Fibroid Registry for Outcomes Data (FIBROID). The purpose of the FIBROID Registry is to assess the procedure's durability, impact on fertility, and quality of life, and to obtain data that will allow researchers to compare UAE to other fibroid therapies. In addition, it will facilitate long-term surveillance of patients undergoing the procedure. The registry will provide physicians and their patients with additional information to allow more informed decision-making regarding the treatment of fibroids.

Secondary objectives of the registry include: measuring the number of patients undergoing UAE; assessing and benchmarking clinical practice patterns (patient selection, technique, use of procedure across country); and collecting and quantifying resource utilization of patients undergoing UAE. A concise set of baseline, short- and long-term functional and clinical outcome data for patients undergoing UAE is being collected to achieve the registry objectives. Patient characteristics, procedural data, in-hospital events, and post-discharge events (to 30-days) are being collected on all patients. Longitudinal data greater than 30-days is being collected from approximately 25 high-volume sites and includes follow-up at 6, 12, and 24 months for assessment of clinical outcomes, quality of life, and patient satisfaction. In addition, all consented patients intending subsequent pregnancy are assessed for fertility and pregnancy history during these periodic contacts. Funding is being sought to continue longitudinal follow-up to five years. Over 1700 cases were enrolled in the registry by 42 sites during the first year.

Quality of life is being measured in the registry by a disease-specific quality-of-life instrument for fibroids. The uterine-fibroid symptom and health-related quality-of-Life (UFS-QOL) questionnaire has been validated and is able to discriminate between normal women and women with uterine fibroids, as well as detect varying signs of symptom severity and symptom impact on quality of life.[15] The questionnaire asks about symptoms experienced by women who have uterine fibroids as well as women's feelings and experiences regarding the impact of uterine fibroid symptoms on their life. The UFS-QOL is available through CIRREF for use in other research studies. The investigators hope that the instruments used in the FIBROID Registry will be used for similar studies of other current and emerging fibroid therapies to allow useful comparison of patient cohorts.

Current status

UAE for the treatment of symptomatic fibroids was first performed in the United States in 1996. Since that time, there has been exponential growth. During 2000 alone, over 4500 procedures were performed in the United States, which is greater than the aggregate experience of the first four years.[16] It is difficult to gauge the actual aggregate volume of this procedure. SIR conducted two surveys in 1999 and 2000 to gain a better understanding of the volume of this pro-

cedure. As of September 2000, there were 10 500 procedures documented in the world.[16] Data from the surveys provide a lower bound to the actual number of procedures performed. It is estimated that at least 20 000 to 25 000 procedures have been performed in the world with the majority performed in the United States. It is also worth noting the rapid diffusion of this procedure from academic to non-academic settings as well as geographically, as UAE is currently being performed in at least 47 states and in the District of Columbia. UAE is also being performed throughout Europe, Asia, South America, and Australia.

Competing technologies

There have been several reports of other procedures that purport to control fibroid symptoms by occluding the main segments of the uterine arteries.[17–19] These laparoscopic procedures have several obvious disadvantages. First, they require general anesthesia and invasion of the peritoneal cavity when compared to UAE. It is unclear whether the equivalent of a proximal embolization will durably devascularize the fibroid microvasculature, as happens during UAE. Finally, obliteration of the proximal segment of the uterine artery by ligation or cautery does not leave access to the uterine vascular bed for repeat embolization in case of procedure failure or fibroid recurrence. For these reasons the authors feel that these procedures will not become as popular as UAE, which is less invasive, involves durable distal embolization of the peri-fibroid vascular bed, and is repeatable if necessary.

Supply and demand

Many women with symptomatic fibroids are told that hysterectomy is their only option despite the general availability of uterus-sparing procedures such as myomectomy and UAE. This appears to be particularly true for African-American women, who have a higher hysterectomy rate than Caucasian women. Women's interest in UAE has been very strong. Women are looking for alternatives to hysterectomy that allow them to keep their bodies intact while alleviating debilitating symptoms. In addition, women are very interested in returning to work as soon as possible after an intervention. Modern life is increasingly busy and most women do not want or are unable to take six weeks to recuperate from a hysterectomy. Women want to get better with the least amount of interruption in their daily lives.

Women are proactively seeking UAE as a treatment option. Many women have referred themselves directly to interventional radiologists for initial evaluation and the procedure. To date, demand for UAE has been largely patient-driven.

The advent of the internet has facilitated the advancement of this procedure and referrals for it. There are numerous on-line chat groups and web sites dedicated to this procedure as well as support groups designed specifically for women with fibroids. Sixty-six percent of all adults in the United States are online of whom 51% are female.[20] Hence, the internet has served as a conduit for those interested in learning more about fibroids and their treatment options.

Major media coverage and the proliferation of web sites have provided information to the medical consumer and have created demand. The rapid growth of UAE signifies the high level of consumer interest for minimally invasive procedures. It is anticipated that the demand for UAE will increase as it becomes more widespread and accepted as the standard of care.

In order to gauge the potential demand for UAE, the reader is invited to consider the following estimate. Assume a medium-sized American urban area with a population of about 4 000 000 people. Half (2 000 000) are female. Approximately 25% (500 000) of those females are within the current target age range for UAE (30–50 years). Assuming that approximately 40% of those women have fibroids, and that 50% of those with fibroids are symptomatic, one can estimate a patient population of roughly 100 000 women with fibroid disease and symptoms justifying treatment. If 50% of women who have symptomatic fibroids are candidates for UAE, then the potential patient population for UAE in that area is approximately 50 000.

A single interventional radiologist whose practice is dedicated to UAE can probably treat 400–500 women annually. An interventional radiologist with a general interventional radiology (IR) practice can probably treat no more than 100–150 women per year. Assuming that the numbers of women treatable by a practicing gynecologist are similar, it is clear that the number of potential patients exceeds the capacity of the available medical personnel.

Currently there is a shortage of interventional radiologists to meet the current demand for their services. With the anticipated growth of UAE this will create further demand on the interventionalist's time. Some IR practices in the United States currently have a waiting list for UAE consultation and procedure appointments. As this procedure continues to be adopted by more interventionalists the waiting times may go down somewhat, but there will never be enough interventional radiologist time available to meet all of the demand.

The currently accepted indications for UAE are the presence of bleeding and/or bulk-related symptoms due to fibroids in the absence of other significant pelvic pathology. There are several issues that, if resolved, may increase the potential applicability of UAE.

There are several reports of successful pregnancies after UAE.[21–24] In addition, the available historical data suggests that fertility is preserved in women who have had both UAE for other indications[25,26] and in women who have had surgical devascularization of the uterus.[27,28] As more data is gathered, it appears that UAE may well prove to be a good option for at least some women with fibroid disease and subfertility. This is especially attractive for women with multiple fibroids, in whom the risk of complications of myomectomy may be higher than for those with single or few fibroids.

There are at least some women who continue to have symptomatic fibroids even after menopause, especially while on hormone replacement therapy (HRT). Women who have vaginal bleeding after menopause must be carefully evaluated for the presence of endometrial carcinoma, and UAE may not be an appropriate choice in women with this complaint. However, there are potentially many women who have continued bulk-related symptoms from fibroids after the cessation of menses and in the absence of vaginal bleeding. UAE in these women has been reported, with good initial results.[29] If UAE proves to be as useful a therapy for post-menopausal women as it is for pre-menopausal women, the demand for the procedure may rise significantly.

Clinical skill set

The clinical care required for treating a woman with fibroids is a paradigm shift for many radiologists. Most interventional radiology procedures are performed in the angio suite. A commitment to clinical practice is essential. Developing a UAE practice takes time. Time needs to be set aside in an office setting to evaluate patients pre-procedure and to provide routine follow-up care. An initial consultation with the patient is necessary. An IR needs to do the history, answer the woman's questions, and ensure she has had a thorough pre-procedure evaluation, including a recent pelvic examination and a current Pap (Papanicolaou) smear. Referral letters need to be provided back to the gynecologist or other referring physician on an ongoing basis, and staff have to be provided to manage patient flow and practice business issues.

There have been some efforts to develop pathways where gynecologists can "learn to do" UAE. These are unrealistic. Embolotherapy is a core portion of the skill set of interventional radiologists, one that is not shared by any other medical specialty. In order to properly perform embolotherapy procedures such as UAE, the operating physician must have extensive skills in diagnostic and therapeutic angiography, which require extensive training. This allows the interventional radiologist to perform this procedure with the high success rates (both technical and clinical) and low complication rates that are expected according to published standards.[30,32]

There are physicians who perform vascular interventions after meeting lower training requirements than those mentioned above. However, in direct comparison, vascular surgeons have been shown to have procedure failure rate twice that of interventional radiologists with a threefold higher complication rate.[31]

UAE is a complex and challenging procedure. It requires extensive training to be performed with high success rates and patient safety.[32] It is unfeasible from an economic or career standpoint for a non-radiologist to seek the level of training required to achieve expertise comparable to that of an experienced interventional radiologist.

Patient safety and therapeutic success are the only legitimate factors determining who should perform any procedure. Based on previous experience with other interventional procedures,[31] it is unreasonable to expect that any physician group other than interventional radiologists (or those with similar levels of training) can perform UAE with acceptable outcomes.

Future directions

There are a number of issues surrounding UAE that remain to be defined. As we gain more information about fertility and about UAE in post-menopausal women, the indications for the procedure will continue to evolve and have increasing specificity. There are still many questions that must be answered to establish the optimal embolic material to use and the optimal technique for the procedure, as well as development of improved protocols for patient management before and after the procedure itself. The place of UAE in the range of therapies for fibroids will be continually redefined, both in regards to current and conventional therapies and as new therapies are developed.

Summary

It is clear that UAE has emerged as a safe and effective treatment for symptomatic fibroids. With time, it will probably become one of the dominant treatments for fibroid disease. Patient care will be best served by gynecologists and interventional radiologists working together to evaluate and treat patients. This may evolve into a variety of practice models, ranging from individual practices with mutual referral patterns to multispecialty group practices. As these models develop there will be increased patient flow into those practices that offer patients the greatest number of options, and pay close consideration to the desires of individual patients to participate in the decision-making process of their own health care.

REFERENCES

The publisher has used its best endeavors to ensure that the URLs for external websites referred to in this book are correct and active at the time of going to press. However, the publisher has no responsibility for the websites and can make no guarantee that a site will remain live or that the content is or will remain appropriate.

1. Broder MS, Harris K, Morton SC, Sherbourne C & Brook RH (1999). *Uterine Artery Embolization: a Systematic Review of the Literature and Proposal for Research*. Publication MR-1158. Santa Monica, CA: RAND.

2. Ravina JH, Bouret JM, Fried D, et al. (1995). Value of preoperative embolization of uterine fibroma: report of a multicenter series of 31 cases. *Contraception, Fertilitie, Sexualitie* **23**: 45–9.

3. Ravina JH, Herbreteau D, Ciraru-Vigneron N, et al. (1995). Arterial embolisation to treat uterine myomata. *Lancet* **346**: 671–2.

4. Heaston DK, Mineau DE, Brown BJ & Miller FJ (1979). Transcatheter arterial embolization for the control of persistent massive puerperal hemorrhage after bilateral surgical hypogastric artery ligation. *Am J Roentgenol* **133**: 152–4.

5. Oliver JA & Lance JS (1979). Selective embolization to control massive hemorrhage following pelvic surgery. *Am J Obstet Gynecol* **135**: 431–2.

6. Frates MC, Benson CB, Doubilet PM, DiSalvo DN, Brown DL, Laing FC, Rein MS & Osathanondh R (1994). Cervical ectopic pregnancy: results of conservative treatment. *Radiology* **191**: 773–5.

7. Dubois J, Garel L, Grignon A, Lemay M & Leduc L (1997). Placenta percreta: balloon occlusion and embolization of the internal iliac arteries to reduce intraoperative blood losses. *Am J Obstet Gynecol* **176**: 723–6.

8. Hutchins FL, Worthington-Kirsch RL & Berkowitz RP (1999). Selective uterine artery embolization as primary treatment for symptomatic leiomyomata uteri: a review of 305 consecutive cases. *J Am Assoc Gynecol Laparosc* **6**: 279–84.

9. Goodwin SC, McLucas B, Lee M, et al. (1999). Uterine artery embolization for the treatment of uterine leiomyomata: midterm results. *J Vasc Interv Radiol* **10**: 1159–65.

10. Spies JB, Levy EB, Wood BJ & Gomez-Jorge J (2000). Uterine artery embolization of symptomatic leiomyomata: observations on our initial experience at Georgetown University Medical Center. *Seminars in Intervent Radiol* **17**: 255–62.

11. Bruneau L, Herbreteau D, Gallas S, Cottier JP, Lebrun JL, Tranquart F, Fauchier F, Body G & Rouleau P (2000). Uterine artery embolization in the primary treatment of uterine leiomyomas: technical features and prospective follow-up with clinical and sonographic examinations in 58 patients. *Am J Roentgenol* **175**: 1267–72.

12. Spies JB, Ascher S, Roth A, Kim J, Levy EB & Gomez-Jorge J (2001). Uterine artery embolization for leiomyomata. *Obstet & Gynecol* **98**: 29–34.

13. Pinto I (2001). Uterine artery embolization vs. hysterectomy: results of a clinical trial. Presented at *"New Trends in Embolotherapy" CIRSE Satellite Symposium* sponsored by Biosphere Medical, 24 September 2001, Gothenburg, Sweden. (Unpublished abstract.)

14. Spies JB, Cooper JM, Worthington-Kirsch RL, Lipman JC, Benenati JM & McLucas B (2002). Uterine artery embolization (UAE) using embospheres: initial results of a phase II comparative study. *J Vasc Interv Radiol* **13**: S20.

15. Spies JB, Coyne K, Guao N, Boyle D, Skynarz-Murphy K & Gonzalves SM (2002). The UFS-QOL: A new disease-specific symptom and health-related quality of life questionnaire for leiomyomata. *Obstet Gynecol* **99**: 290–300.

16. Landow W (2001). UAE survey results. *SCVIR News* **14**(May/June): col. 3.

17. Forcier N, Altieri G, Jones M & Burbank F (1999). A new alternative to uterine artery embolization. Presented at *The Second International Symposium on the Embolization of Uterine Myomata*, 17–18 September 1999, Boston, MA, USA. (Unpublished abstract.)

18. Lee PI, Chang YK, Yoon JB & Chi YS (1999). Preliminary experience with uterine artery ligation for symptomatic uterine leiomyomas. *J Am Assoc Gynecol Laparosc* **6**: S27–28.

19. Liu WM (2000). Laparoscopic bipolar coagulation of uterine vessels to treat symptomatic leiomyomas. *J Am Assoc Gynecol Laparosc* **7**: 125–9.

20. Taylor H (2002). Internet penetration at 66% of Adults (137 million) nationwide. The Harris Poll® 2002 Apr 17 [cited 2002 May 6]; 18:[1 screen]. Available from URL:

http://www.harrisinteractive.com/harris_poll/index.asp?
PID = 295.

21. Ravina JH, Ciraru-Vigneron N, Aymard A, LeDref O &
Merland JJ (2002). Pregnancy after embolization of uterine
myoma: report of 12 cases. *Fertil Steril* **73**: 1241–3.

22. McLucas B, Goodwin S, Adler L, Rappaport A, Reed R &
Perella R (2001). Pregnancy following uterine artery embolization. *Intl J Gyn Obstet* **74**: 1–7.

23. Sterling KM, Siskin GP, Ponturo MM, Mandato K, Rholl KS &
Cooper JM (2002). A multi-center study evaluating the use
of gelfoam only for uterine artery embolization for symptomatic leiomyomata. *J Vasc Interv Radiol* **13**: S19.

24. Walker WJ & Pelage JP (2002). Uterine fibroid embolisation:
results in 400 women with imaging follow-up. *J Vasc Interv
Radiol* **13**: S18.

25. Stancato-Pasik A, Mitty HA, Richard HM, III & Eshkkar
NS (1996). Obstetric Embolotherapy: Effect on Menses and
Pregnancy. *Radiology* **201**(P): 179.

26. McIvor J & Cameron EW (1996). Pregnancy after uterine
artery embolization to control haemorrhage from gestational trophoblastic disease. *Br J Radiol* **69**: 624–9.

27. Mengert WF, Burchell RC, Blumstein RW & Daskal JL (1969).
Pregnancy after bilateral ligation of the internal iliac and
ovarian arteries. *Obstet Gynecol* **34**: 664–6.

28. Shinagawa S, Nomura Y & Kudoh S (1981). Full-term deliveries after ligation of bilateral internal iliac arteries and
infundibulopelvic ligaments. *Acta Obstet Gynecol Scand* **60**:
439–40.

29. Min RJ, Troiano R, Kandarpa K et al. (2002). Uterine fibroid
embolization in post-menopausal women. *J Vasc Interv
Radiol* **13**: S64.

30. Drooz AT, Lewis CA, Allen TE et al. (1997). Quality improvement guidelines for percutaneous transcatheter embolization. *J Vasc Interv Radiol* **8**: 889–95.

31. Ayoub DM, Muehle CM & Neal CE (1997). Percutaneous endovascular treatment of peripheral vascular disease: outcome differences between interventional radiologists and
vascular surgeons. *J Vasc Interv Radiol* **8**(Suppl 2): 214.

32. Spies J, Niedzwiecki G, Goodwin S et al. (2001). Training stan-
dards for physicians performing uterine artery embolization
for leiomyomata: consensus statement developed by the
Task Force of Uterine Artery Embolization and the Standards
Division of the Society of Cardiovascular & Interventional
Radiology – August 2000. *J Vasc Interv Radiol* **12**: 19–21.

Index